LINGUA PHARMA

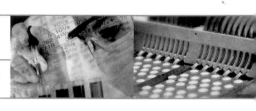

A GLOSSARY OF TERMS FOR THE PHARMACEUTICAL INDUSTRY

JOHN J. CAMPBELL

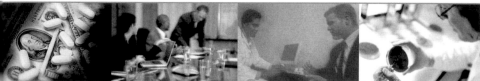

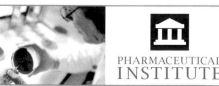

PHARMACEUTICAL
INSTITUTE

Library of Congress Control Number: 2005906560

ISBN 0-9763096-1-0

To learn more about the full range of off-the-shelf and custom information and training resources offered by the Pharmaceutical Institute, visit us online at www.pharmainstitute.com or call (877) 923-5600.

Pharmaceutical Institute
Raleigh, NC 27615

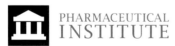

Book design and layout by Susan Wang, www.savantstudio.com

FOREWORD

During my years within and as a consultant to the pharmaceutical and biotech industry, I have had many opportunities to observe a phenomenon that is no doubt as old as humankind—the reluctance to admit to gaps in our understanding.

That reluctance is particularly strong when it concerns the terminology in common currency among our colleagues.

Such embarrassment is absolutely groundless in our industry, when the variety and sheer number of terms are too much for any person, no matter how experienced, to absorb. This embarrassment is also costly, because it inhibits very able people from participating fully in discussions and decision making.

Lingua Pharma is a humble attempt at bridging those gaps. We have tried to produce a more comprehensive glossary of terms than we found elsewhere. We also strove to develop highly practical definitions that readers could readily understand and put to work.

Inevitably, there will be flaws in the book we produced. It is impossible to cover all terms in industry use. It is also impossible to attain universal agreement with the definitions we have provided. Knowing many of these terms are employed differently in different contexts and by different companies, we tried to select the meanings in most common usage.

Lingua Pharma includes our best layman's understanding of certain legal and regulatory terms. We are, of course, not lawyers, and you shouldn't rely on those legal and regulatory definitions in making decisions.

Despite its limitations, we believe *Lingua Pharma* is a valuable reference tool, and hope it will earn a prominent place on your bookshelves. We will continue to improve upon and expand it in the years to come.

John J. Campbell

Chief Executive Officer

Campbell Alliance

GLOSSARY OF TERMS

Warning: Any definitions of regulatory or legal terms are not intended as legal advice. Before taking or refraining from any action, users should seek expert legal counsel on the meaning and implications of such terms.

A

AAHP (American Association of Health Plans)

The primary US association of health plans, which includes health maintenance organizations (HMOs), preferred provider organizations (PPOs), other forms of managed care, and utilization review organizations (UROs).

AA rated

See AB rated.

absorption

The movement of a drug from the site of administration (e.g., mouth) into the blood stream. Absorption of a drug is affected by its chemical properties, its formulation, and its route of administration.

absorption rate

The rate at which a drug is taken into a person's blood stream within a specified time period. Absorption rates can vary wildly from person to person, creating the challenge of refining a drug so that it is effective on people with low absorption rates but not toxic to people with high absorption rates.

AB rated

The designation the FDA accords to drugs considered therapeutically equivalent to a specified brand and therefore appropriate generic substitutes. The first letter (A) signifies therapeutic equivalence and the second (B) signifies the basis upon which therapeutic equivalence was assessed.

AB-rated drugs have proven bioequivalent in human trials, while AA-rated drugs have not been tested in this manner but are considered unlikely to have bioavailability problems.

academic detailing

See counterdetailing.

academic medical center (AMC)

A teaching institution—that is, one that has a medical school, physician residency programs, and the leading-edge specialty programs required to train them.

accelerated approval

A specialized FDA mechanism implemented in the early 1990s to speed approval of drugs that represent a major advance in addressing serious or life-threatening diseases for which no effective alternative treatments exist. The impetus was the demand for new AIDS therapies.

Under accelerated approval, the FDA accepts a surrogate endpoint as evidence of effectiveness, and then requires post-marketing studies to confirm the drug's benefits.

See Fast Track and Priority Review.

access

A patient's ability to obtain needed medical services. Variables related to ease of access include availability of insurance, location of healthcare facilities, convenience of operating hours, and service cost. See reimbursement and access.

account

An institutional customer assigned to a Managed Markets account manager. The account may be an MCO, a federal customer such as the Department of Defense or the Veterans Health Administration, a retail pharmacy chain, a hospital, a pharmacy benefits manager (PBM), or an employer.

account managers

Managed Markets personnel charged with calling on important institutional customers (payers, pharmacy benefits management companies, providers such as hospitals, and employers) and obtaining access for their company's drugs.

ACE inhibitors

Angiotensin-converting enzyme inhibitors. A class of drugs used to treat cardiovascular conditions such as hypertension and chronic heart failure.

action letter

The FDA's official response to an NDA (an action letter is also known as an NDA action). The message may be an approval letter, approvable letter, or a non-approvable letter.

active control group

In a clinical trial a group of participants who receive an active comparator drug as opposed to a placebo or the investigational/study drug (see treatment arm)

active ingredient

See API.

activities of daily living (ADL)

Activities that the average person can perform autonomously, such as walking, getting in and out of bed, dressing, bathing, eating, and using the bathroom. A person's ability to perform these functions unaided is a measure of health status and dependency.

actual acquisition cost (AAC)

The net cost to a particular pharmacy of purchasing a drug, taking into account discounts, rebates, chargebacks and other adjustments.

For larger pharmacy chains with purchasing clout, AAC is often considerably less than the average wholesale price, or AWP. In order to be equitable to pharmacies that buy drugs at different price points, payers sometimes try to determine actual cost and reimburse that plus a dispensing fee.

acuity (patient acuity)

Measurement of the intensity of care required for a patient provided by a registered nurse. There are six categories ranging from minimal care to intensive care.

acute

In terms of diseases or conditions, abrupt in onset and short-term (as opposed to chronic).

acute care

Short-term medical treatment, usually in a hospital or an urgent care center, for patients having an acute illness or injury or recovering from surgery.

acute illness

A condition or illness that only lasts for a short period of time. The common cold is an acute illness.

ad board

See advisory board.

adherence

Taking a drug exactly as prescribed.

adjuvant

A substance that enhances the action of a drug or antigen. Adjuvant therapy is the use of a second form of treatment in addition to the primary therapy, for example, having chemotherapy in addition to surgery or radiation therapy.

ADME

An acronym for absorption, distribution, metabolism, and excretion. Tests performed to assess the impact of a drug on the human body (sometimes referred to as pharmacokinetics). The ideal product will be rapidly absorbed, distributed to the target organ, broken down (metabolized) efficiently without generating any toxic substances, and excreted effectively from the body without harming the kidneys or other organs.

ADMET

ADME testing combined with toxicology testing.

adulterant

A substance that lessens the purity or effectiveness of a drug—also known as a contaminant.

advanced practice nurse

An umbrella term given to a registered nurse who has met advanced educational and clinical practice requirements beyond the two to four years of basic nursing education required for all RNs.

adverse drug reaction (ADR)

An unwanted, negative consequence sometimes associated with the use of drug therapy. It is a more precise term than "side effect," as some side effects may be therapeutically useful. Other synonyms are "adverse effects" and "adverse events."

adverse effect

See adverse drug reaction.

adverse event

Undesirable or unexpected occurrence affecting the health of patients or clinical trial participants while they are taking a medication. The term includes both occurrences that are known or suspected to be related to drug use and those that have no causal relation. For instance, in a clinical trial, both a headache and a car accident would be considered adverse events, although only the former is likely to be causally related to the drug under scrutiny.

adverse event form

Document for capturing all adverse events related to a clinical trial or a marketed product.

adverse event reporting

Reports to regulators of serious and unexpected adverse events during clinical trials and once a product is on the market. The FDA has established an Adverse Event Reporting System (AERS)—a computerized information database designed for use in post-marketing surveillance of the safety of approved drugs and therapeutic biologic products. Manufacturers are required to participate in the AERS, and healthcare professionals and consumers participate voluntarily through the MedWatch program.

advertising

In the pharmaceutical context, traditional paid promotions appearing in various media. Advertisements enumerated in the Federal Food, Drug and Cosmetic Act of 1938 include print ads (in published journals, magazines, other periodicals, and newspapers) and broadcasts through media such as radio, television, and telephone communication systems. The FDA also regulates a broader category of communications known as promotions.

advisory board

In the pharmaceutical context, a focus group (often consisting of payers and/ or physicians) convened by a pharmaceutical company to obtain expert input on such issues as the probable reception of a product approaching launch. Also called an ad board.

affinity

The extent to which a drug binds to its intended target (e.g., a receptor or enzyme).

Agency for Healthcare Research and Quality (AHRQ)

An agency within the US Public Health Service responsible for research on the quality, appropriateness, effectiveness, and cost of healthcare. Formerly the Agency for Health Care Policy and Research (AHCPR).

agonists

Drugs that achieve their beneficial effect by binding with a receptor and producing a response that mimics or enhances normal cell functions.

AHA (American Hospital Association)

A national association that represents hospitals in the United States; based in Washington, DC.

AIM

Active ingredient manufacturer.

alignment

The manner in which client responsibilities are allocated among sales representatives in a pharmaceutical company—e.g., by therapeutic area and/or by geography, as well as by sales potential of a given assignment.

allele

One of the forms that a gene at a particular location on a chromosome can take. Differences in alleles are responsible for differences in inherited characteristics, such as hair color and blood type.

allied health personnel

Specially trained and often licensed health workers other than physicians, dentists, optometrists, chiropractors, podiatrists, and nurses.

ALF

See assisted living facility.

ALOS

Average length of stay. Typically in reference to hospitalization duration.

AMA (American Medical Association)

A national association based in Chicago that represents more than 700,000 medical doctors in the United States. Among other things, the AMA defines ethical standards that physicians should observe in their relationships with pharmaceutical companies and in their prescribing behavior.

ambulatory care

Any health service that does not require an inpatient stay—including physical therapy, physician office visits, ER visits, outpatient surgery, and home healthcare.

ambulatory surgery center (ASC)

An outpatient surgery site for patients who do not require post-procedure hospitalization. It may be located on a hospital campus or at a convenient stand-alone site.

AMCP (Academy of Managed Care Pharmacy)

An organization for pharmacy directors. The AMCP is the national professional society dedicated to pharmaceutical care in managed healthcare environments.

American Pharmaceutical Association (APhA)

The national professional society of pharmacists, founded in 1852; it was the first and is still the largest professional association of pharmacists in the United States. The members of APhA include practicing pharmacists, pharmaceutical scientists, pharmacy students, and pharmacy technicians.

amino acids

Any of a class of 20 molecules that are the building blocks of proteins in living things. The sequence of amino acids in a protein, and its function, are determined by genetic code.

AMP

See average manufacturer's price.

amplification

In genetic research, the process of copying DNA fragments to increase the supply available for testing and study.

ampoule or ampule

A small glass vial that is sealed after being filled and is chiefly used as a container for a hypodermic injection solution.

analogs or analogues

In a commercial context, a marketed drug whose similarities to a product in development make it a useful comparator for purposes of assessing market potential and planning market strategy.

In a clinical context, a drug that is very similar to another compound but differs slightly in chemical structure.

ancillary care

Supplemental health services that facilitate diagnosis and treatment, including lab work and x-rays.

ANDA (Abbreviated New Drug Application)

An application to the FDA for approval of a generic drug that is bioequivalent to a brand whose patent has expired.

The process is abbreviated because the generic manufacturer is generally allowed to rely on safety and efficacy data from the brand manufacturer's New Drug Application (NDA). Instead of conducting preclinical and clinical trials, the generic manufacturer must scientifically demonstrate that its product is bioequivalent. The ANDA system, which was introduced in 1984 in the Hatch-Waxman Act, has allowed many generics companies to have a drug ready to market when the patent of the drug with the same active ingredient expires.

antagonists

A chemical substance that interferes with the physiological action of another, especially by combining with and blocking its nerve receptor.

antibiotics

A substance produced by or derived from certain fungi, bacteria, and other organisms, that can destroy or inhibit the growth of other microorganisms. Penicillin is an example.

antibodies

The body's protective mechanism for warding off infection and disease. Antibodies are proteins produced by the immune system in response to foreign substances (antigens). Each antibody binds a specific antigen that is its structural complement in order to neutralize the antigen.

antigens

Any foreign substance that, when introduced into the body, causes the immune system to create an antibody to fight or destroy it. Examples include toxins, bacteria, foreign blood cells, and the cells of transplanted organs.

antimicrobial agents

Agents that kill disease-causing microbes (micro-organisms). Categories of such agents include antiviral, antibacterial, antifungal, and antiparasitic drugs.

anti-infectives

A therapeutic area covering drugs that fight infections in the body caused by micro-organisms. Also another name for antimicrobial agents.

anti-kickback laws

Laws that bar pharmaceutical companies and other entities from giving physicians or other healthcare providers money or other economic inducements to encourage utilization of their products. At the federal level, the Medicare and Medicaid Protection Act of 1987 is known as the anti-kickback statute.

antisense drugs

Drugs whose purpose is to switch off the production of disease-causing proteins. The strands of genetic material that contain the instructions for generation of these proteins are called "sense" strands.

APCs (ambulatory payment classifications)

The coding system under which Medicare pays for outpatient hospital services. Services in each APC are similar clinically in terms of the resources they require. A payment rate is established for each APC. Depending on the services provided, hospitals may be paid for more than one APC in a single encounter.

API (active pharmaceutical ingredient)

The part of a drug formulation that is responsible for achieving a therapeutic effect. Also known as the drug substance or the active ingredient.

APLB (Advertising and Promotional Labeling Branch)

The branch of the FDA that regulates promotions of most biologics (and is, therefore, part of CBER). It is to biologics what the Division of Drug Marketing, Advertising and Communications (see DDMAC) is to chemical drugs. Its duties include identification of false or misleading promotional materials.

applicant

In the context of FDA processes, a drug sponsor.

approvable letter

An FDA response to an NDA that lists minor issues to be resolved before marketing approval can be granted.

approval letter

An FDA response to an NDA that grants permission to market a drug in the US. A product can be legally marketed in the US on the day a division or office director from the FDA signs an approval letter.

arm

See treatment arm.

assay

A lab test to assess such drug characteristics as composition, purity, and potency (level of biologic or chemical activity). Its primary purpose is to determine which substances—and how much of each—are in a sample.

ASHP (American Society of Health-System Pharmacists)

The national professional organization for pharmacists who work in hospitals, HMOs, long-term care facilities, home care, and other components of the healthcare system.

ASO (administrative services only) agreement

A contract under which a self-insured employer that has retained the financial responsibility for covering healthcare claims from its employees hires a third party (ASO) to administer those payments. Administrative services include claims adjudication, member services, and management information reporting. ASO is also used to refer to the entities providing such services.

assisted living facility (ALF)

Programs offered in a residential community to support the infirm elderly or others who need ongoing monitoring and support to ensure their continued well-being. Typical services include meals, laundry, housekeeping, medication reminders, and assistance with activities of daily living (ADLs). Assisted living facilities usually provide less intensive care than skilled nursing facilities (and, therefore, are not appropriate for patients with extremely severe or complex health problems).

atom

The smallest possible component of an element.

authorization

The advance approval of some form of treatment, including use of a specified prescription drug. Under managed care, authorization of expensive resources is often a prerequisite for reimbursement (see prior authorization).

authorized generic

The generic product of a company that has purchased licensing rights from the owner of the original brand-name ethical product.

autoimmune disease

A condition, such as lupus, in which the immune system mistakenly attacks the body's own organs and tissues.

autosomes

Any chromosomes other than those that determine sex. Human cells have 22 pairs of autosomes.

average manufacturer's price (AMP)

The average payment a manufacturer receives, after discounts, from a wholesaler for drugs that are then distributed to retail pharmacies. This price is used to calculate the rebates due to Medicaid programs, which are entitled to a rate lower than AWP.

average wholesale price (AWP)

A national average of list prices charged by wholesalers to pharmacies. Although the AWP is supposed to reflect the sum pharmacies pay wholesalers for the drugs they sell, in reality it is often more like a "sticker price"—considerably higher than the actual price that larger purchasers (e.g., major retail pharmacy chains) normally pay.

B

bacteria
Single-cell organisms that can sometimes cause infections, such as strep throat and bacterial pneumonia.

base pairs
The building blocks of genes, which are made of four substances: adenine (A), guanine (G), cytosine (C), and thymine (T). Each human being has billions of base pairs.

batch
A specified quantity of a drug substance produced in a single manufacturing cycle and expected to be homogeneous.

batch records
The road map for manufacturing a batch of a product and the documentation filled out for each batch manufactured.

A master production batch record (MPBR) is a step-by-step description of the entire production process for a specific drug. It ensures compliance with the fundamentals of cGMP and provides practical instructions for the manufacturing team. The MPBR explains exactly how the product is produced, what raw materials are to be used, and how quality controls should be executed.

B cells
White blood cells that develop in the bone marrow and are the source of antibodies. Also known as B lymphocytes.

behind-the-counter drugs

Drugs that do not require a prescription but are sufficiently strong or subject to abuse that they are not available on retail pharmacy shelves; they must be requested from and provided by a pharmacist.

The decision to make a drug a behind-the-counter product is generally left to each pharmacy. Pain relievers or cough medicines that include codeine are sometimes included in this category, as are drugs that can be used to manufacture methamphetamines.

bench work

Laboratory research

best price

The requirement that Medicaid and some other government customers receive the lowest prices that a pharmaceutical company offers on each of its products.

Under the Social Security Act, the term "best price" for a brand or generic is the lowest price available from the relevant pharmaceutical company during the rebate period to any wholesaler, retailer, provider, health maintenance organization, nonprofit entity, or governmental entity in the US during the relevant time period. For purposes of determining Medicaid rebates, prices paid for drugs by a number of federal and state entities, such the Veterans Health Administration, are excluded from "best price" analysis.

Big 4

The four largest purchasers of pharmaceuticals within the federal government: the Department of Veterans Affairs (VA), Department of Defense, Public Health Service, and Coast Guard. Like all federal agencies, these four have the right to purchase pharmaceuticals from the federal supply schedule-but they are often eligible for prices below FSS on brand-name drugs, which are subject to a federal ceiling price.

Big Pharma

A term for the global pharmaceutical industry, usually used in reference to the top 10 to 20 global research-based drug manufacturers.

BIND (biologic investigational new drug)
An IND submitted for a biologic.

BIO (Biotechnology Industry Organization)
A trade association that represents biotechnology firms.

bioavailability
The amount of an active ingredient that reaches the drug target and remains in the body for a sufficient time to have a therapeutic effect–and the rate at which it reaches that target.

To obtain FDA marketing approval, generics manufacturers must prove, among other things, that their product's bioavailability is equivalent to that of a specified brand when administered in equal doses under similar conditions. See bioequivalence.

bioequivalence
The standard that a generic must meet in order to win FDA marketing approval. Bioequivalence is established by comparison to a branded ethical drug. Two bioequivalent, drugs, using equal amounts of the same active ingredient, will produce the same concentration in blood and tissues when administered in identical treatment regimens. Drugs that are bioequivalent are assumed to be therapeutically equivalent–that is, to have the same therapeutic effect and toxicity profile.

bioinformatics
The collection, organization, and analysis of large amounts of biological information using sophisticated computer techniques. Often mentioned in the context of genomics research, which requires the management of huge stores of data.

biological products or biologics
Drugs, blood, and blood products manufactured through a biological process and derived from living sources (humans, animals, plants, and microorganisms), rather than through the chemical synthesis by which most drugs are created. The most common form of biologic is the vaccine. Within the FDA, most biologics are regulated by CBER (Center for Biologics Evaluation and Research). See large molecules.

biopharmaceuticals

Drugs derived from biologic sources.

biotechnology

The use of biological processes (that is, the manipulation of living organisms) to develop or manufacture such products as drugs (including vaccines). Biotechnology holds out the promise of drugs tailored to a person's specific genetic makeup.

biotechs

Firms that focus on the development of biologics and/or technologies to support biologic research. Using life science technologies, they hope to discover and develop marketable new medicines. Most of these firms are research-side-only enterprises that seek outside partners for commercialization..

BLA (biologic license application)

The special application to the FDA for approval of biologic compounds.

black box warning

The most severe health-risk warning that the FDA can require on the package insert and is displayed in a prominent box. Reserved for drugs that the FDA considers sufficiently beneficial to remain on the market but have serious or life-threatening risks.

blinding or blind study

A clinical trial design in which patients (in the case of single-blind studies) or patients and all the study staff (in the case of double-blind studies) are "kept in the dark" as to who is receiving the investigational drug and who the control drug (placebo or another therapy). The goal is to avoid bias in reporting and assessing results.

blister pack

A form of drug packaging in which pills or capsules are encased in individual plastic pods, which are all attached to a common aluminum-like backing. Users push the plastic pods to extract pills individually through the backing.

blockbuster drugs

Pharmaceuticals in the highest echelon of sales revenue, which bring in $1 billion or more per year in gross revenues.

Blue Book

The generic name for a widely used pharmaceutical pricing guide formally named the American Druggist First Databank Annual Directory of Pharmaceuticals. The Blue Book is intended to represent an average of wholesalers' catalog or list prices for a drug product to their customers (i.e., retailers, hospitals, physicians and other buying entities). Other pricing guides are the Red Book and Medispan's Pricing Guide.

board-certified physician

A physician who has passed an examination administered by a medical specialty board requiring expert knowledge in a particular area of medical practice. The American Board of Medical Specialties in the US certifies physicians in 24 specialties, including allergy and immunology, anesthesiology, dermatology, family practice, medical genetics, preventive medicine, and surgery.

board certification

The testing required to become a board-certified physician.

brand or brand name

A drug product given a catchy proprietary name for promotional purposes, such as Allegra, Viagra, or Sominex. Brands usually are or once were patented ethical products, but, increasingly, generics are also being branded for promotional purposes. Brands can be either OTC or prescription. For an equivalent term, see trade name.

Within pharmaceutical companies, Brand is also sometimes used as shorthand for Brand Management and Marketing.

brand director

The manager responsible for strategy, promotional mix, and profit-and-loss performance of a specific product brand or indication.

Brand Management and Marketing

The pharmaceutical function charged with devising and implementing a commercial and promotional strategy for one or more drug products.

branded ethical products

Brand-name prescription drugs that are or were once under patent.

branded generics

A generic drug that the manufacturer gives a proprietary name for promotional purposes. Motrin is a branded generic. Ibuprofen (the chemical name) is the term for its unbranded equivalent. Typically, the manufacturer is able to charge a higher price for the branded generic by distinguishing its quality, dosage form, or brand name over its unbranded equivalents.

brief summary

Information that the Federal Food, Drug, and Cosmetic Act requires in nearly every advertisement for a drug (whether to consumers or physicians). The brief summary covers side effects, contraindications, and effectiveness. In many advertisements, including most television commercials, manufacturers opt to run "reminder" ads or "help-seeking" ads, both of which are exempt from the brief summary requirement.

bundling or bundled payment

A single payment for a group of related services-for instance, an episode of hospital care.

Business Development (BD)

In the pharmaceutical industry, the function charged with identifying compounds or products for in-licensing or out-licensing and evaluating their risks and value.

C

CAC (Carrier Advisory Committee)

A panel of local physicians who advise Medicare fiscal administrators (the intermediaries who process claims) as to whether they should cover a certain outpatient drug.

CADD (computer-assisted drug design)

The use of computer techniques to discover and optimize drugs.

candidate compound

Compound selected from a group of chemically related options that appears to have the greatest efficacy and fewest side effects. This compound will be the subject of additional screening to assess its viability as a drug.

capitation

Term derived from "per capita"-per head. Advance payments to MCOs (and, in some markets, providers-especially primary care physicians) based on the anticipated cost of health services for a group of enrollees in a health plan. These fees are typically calculated as a flat rate per member per month (PMPM) and do not vary based on the actual services provided to each member. The MCO or physician is at financial risk if the actual costs of care prove higher than the projected costs.

carriers

See Medicare carriers.

carve-out

In the pharmaceutical context, separate management of a specific healthcare benefit, such as outpatient pharmaceutical coverage. The entity overseeing a pharmaceutical carve-out is typically a PBM.

case management

Close supervision by healthcare professionals (usually nurses) of the services provided to and health status of patients with expensive, unpredictable treatment needs (such as those with catastrophic illnesses, multiple diseases, or mental health problems).

CBER (Center for Biologics Evaluation and Research)

The arm of the FDA concerned with regulation of most biologic products. The mission stated on its Web page is "to protect and enhance the public health through regulation of biological products including blood, vaccines, therapeutics, and related drugs and devices, according to statutory authorities."

CDC (Centers for Disease Control and Prevention)

A part of the US Department of Health and Human Services, recognized as the lead federal agency for protecting the health and safety of Americans at home and abroad through programs addressing disease prevention and control, environmental health, and health education.

CDER (Center for Drug Evaluation and Research)

The unit of the FDA with responsibility for oversight of all non-biologic drugs and selected biologics (including monoclonal antibodies, enzymes, growth factors, and proteins). CDER approves such drugs for clinical trials, sets drug manufacturing standards, approves drugs for US marketing, reviews drug labeling and promotions, and monitors marketed drugs for unexpected or severe health risks.

cell

The fundamental self-contained unit of life. In complex organisms, such as humans, cells are the building blocks of different organs and tissues, each charged with particular specialized tasks. Every human cell (except for blood cells) houses the entire genome-all the genetic information necessary to create a human being.

CenterWatch

A widely read clinical development publication.

CFR (Code of Federal Regulations)

The repository for regulations governing the conduct of federal executive departments and agencies, including the FDA. Title 21 of the CFR contains FDA regulations relevant to drug development and manufacturing. When regulations are first produced, they appear in the Federal Register, which is the federal government's "daily awareness publication."

cGMP (Current Good Manufacturing Practices)

See GMP.

channel

A means or medium of outreach to pharmaceutical customers, such as sales representative visits to physicians, TV and print ads, peer-reviewed journal articles, and Web sites.

chargeback

Pricing administration technique in which money is returned by a pharmaceutical company to a wholesaler.

The difference between the price a wholesaler pays a manufacturer (WAC) and the price the wholesaler will charge its own customers, including hospitals. The manufacturer, who is relying on the wholesaler to administer volume discounts to hospitals and other drug purchasers, will pay the wholesaler a rebate-the chargeback-to make up the loss the wholesaler realizes from selling at a lower price that it paid.

chemical name

The (typically lengthy) name assigned to a product based on its underlying chemical structure. For instance, 2-(4-isobutylphenyl)-propionic acid is the chemical name for ibuprofen (see generic name).

chromosomes

Structures found in the nucleus of a cell. Chromosomes, which come in pairs, can be thought of as linked groups of genes that are inherited as a package. A normal human cell contains 46 chromosomes-22 pairs of autosomes and 2 sex chromosomes, X and Y. Each of the 46 human chromosomes contains the DNA for hundreds of individual genes.

chronic condition or disease

Conditions or illnesses that are ongoing or recurring. Chronic diseases can be alleviated, but generally not cured, and therefore involve long-term treatment. Examples include arthritis, multiple sclerosis, and asthma.

chronic therapy or care

Treatment for health problems that are long-term and continuing. Rehabilitation facilities, nursing homes, and mental hospitals are chronic care facilities.

class of trade

A means of segmenting Trade customers (pharmacies and wholesalers), which indicates the type of customer they represent and possibly their eligibility for special contract pricing.

clinic

A treatment facility that provides emergency treatment and ambulatory (out-patient) services, including physical examinations and immunizations. Some clinics also offer rehab services (occupational therapy and physical therapy).

clinical data repository

A collection of medical records (typically computerized) containing inpatient and outpatient histories of a group of patients. These data are useful in treating those patients and, in the aggregate, the records are valuable for clinical research regarding the outcomes of various treatments.

clinical hold

The mechanism that the FDA uses when it is concerned that a study may pose an unreasonable risk to subjects. CDER may either delay the start of an early-phase trial on the basis of information in the IND, or stop an ongoing study. The sponsor must address the problems triggering the hold before the order will be lifted.

clinical investigators

Professionals (usually physicians) charged with overseeing the administration of an experimental compound in clinical trials. Also referred to simply as investigators. The investigator in charge at a site is known as the principal investigator.

clinical practice guidelines or pathways

Summaries of the current medical knowledge about a disease, accompanied by step-by-step process flows that help caregivers make appropriate diagnostic and treatment choices. They often recommend a specific therapeutic category of drugs as a treatment but rarely single out a particular brand. This term is a synonym for critical path.

clinical protocol

A detailed roadmap for conducting and assessing the results of a specific clinical trial, which must be approved by an institutional review board.

As part of the IND submitted to the FDA before clinical trials begin, pharmaceutical companies provide protocols that include number of patients, inclusion and exclusion criteria, proposed treatment regimen, route of drug administration, proposed dosing levels, qualifications of the clinical investigators, proposed study sites, descriptions of the drug's makeup and manufacturing, and a methodology for analyzing study data.

clinical rationale

A medical explanation or scientific hypothesis of how and/or why a drug or treatment regimen works, usually to improve human health. The FDA requires a discussion of the clinical rationale for a drug as part of a pharmaceutical company's NDA filing. See also scientific rationale.

clinical reviewers

See medical reviewers.

clinical trial

The systematic investigation of the effects of a drug, medical treatment, or device on a group of subjects. Clinical trials or studies are used to establish optimal dosing levels, as well as drug safety and efficacy.

clinicians

Healthcare professionals, such as physicians or nurses, who specialize in treating patients rather than, for instance, in conducting experimental medical research.

close

The conclusion of a sales detail, during which the pharmaceutical company sales rep is supposed to ask the prescriber on whom he or she is calling to adopt a specific product.

closed formulary

A formulary with a small list of drugs from which physicians can choose. Some MCOs and PBMs with closed formularies offer (less generous) reimbursement for non-formulary items, but others do not provide any coverage outside the formulary.

closed-model pharmacy

Pharmacies that dispense drugs only to specific populations. For instance, hospital/nursing home pharmacies that provide drugs solely to their patients or HMO pharmacies that only dispense to plan enrollees.

CMC (Chemistry, Manufacturing, and Controls)

The section of a BLA or NDA that describes drug product composition and the proposed drug manufacturing process.

CME (continuing medical education)

Programs to support ongoing learning among physicians, pharmacists, nurses, and other healthcare professionals. As a condition of licensure, physicians must regularly attend a certain number of approved courses or conferences. Pharmaceutical companies sometimes help subsidize such programs.

CMO (contract manufacturing organization)

Entities to which pharmaceutical companies delegate drug manufacture. Both the relatively low-volume manufacture required for pre-clinical and clinical trials and full-scale commercial manufacturing of products approved for marketing may be outsourced to CMOs.

CMS (Centers for Medicare and Medicaid Services)

New name (as of 2001) for the former Health Care Financing Administration (HCFA). The federal regulatory agency charged with administering (and setting rules for) Medicare, as well as overseeing state management of Medicaid. Among other responsibilities, CMS is in charge of creating the security and privacy regulations that were mandated by HIPAA.

co-development (or cooperative development)

A licensing arrangement in which a research-focused company without the funds or resources to complete product development receives a capital infusion from another pharmaceutical company. In exchange, that pharmaceutical company typically receives the "right of first refusal" on compound co-promotion or acquisition.

coding systems

Systems employed in healthcare for grouping similar case types. These categories are used to determine appropriate reimbursement and/or track the clinical efficacy of treatments for patients with similar disorders. For examples, see CPT, DRG, and ICD-9. Coders usually work in medical records departments and coding is a function of billing.

COGS

Cost of goods sold (for accounting and financial statements).

co-insurance

The percentage of the cost of a health product or service for which an insured patient is responsible. Unlike co-payments, which are flat fees regardless of total cost, co-insurance payments vary with the expense of the health product or service.

co-marketing (or cooperative marketing)

A licensing agreement under which two companies sell the same drug in the same market or territory under two different brand names.

combination product

A term encompassing multiple types:

- A single product that includes two or more components that are subject to regulation by the FDA-a drug and device; a biologic and device; or a drug, device, and biologic–that are combined or mixed or produced as a single entity.
- Two or more FDA-regulated products that are packaged and sold together as a unit.
- A drug, device, or biologic that is packaged as a stand–alone but whose labeling or intended use requires another drug, biologic, or device.

combinatorial chemistry

A relatively new science that allows rapid production of thousands of similar molecules (candidate compounds) with slight differences that may affect their efficacy as drugs. In the past, scientists had to develop one molecule at a time, which slowed drug development. Now, millions of similar compounds can be screened against an intended target to identify the best (most effective) one. See high-throughput screening.

commercial INDs

IND applications that are submitted by companies whose ultimate goal is to obtain marketing approval for a new product. The vast majority of INDs, however, are filed for noncommercial research. These noncommercial INDs include Investigator INDs, Emergency Use INDs, and Treatment INDs.

comorbid condition or comorbidity

Health problems in addition to a patient's primary diagnosis (or, in a clinical trial, the disease/condition for which a treatment is being evaluated).

community-based physician

A non–hospital–based, private practice physician.

community hospital

Hospitals, usually unaffiliated with an academic institution or teaching facility, offering medical and surgical care–and sometimes even highly specialized services (e.g., a cardiac unit or radiation oncology)–to the local population.

comparator drug

An investigational or marketed drug (i.e., active control) or placebo used as a reference in a clinical trial.

Compassionate IND

Emergency Use and Treatment INDs, granted by the FDA to speed investigational drugs to populations in urgent need of them (although the term "compassionate" does not appear in the IND regulations). Drugs that are still in clinical testing (investigational drugs) are made available to the physicians of desperately ill or dying patients who are not participating in the clinical studies. Sometimes referred to as compassionate use.

compliance

The extent to which a patient follows the regimen ordered by his/her physician during a designated time frame (e.g., the observation period of a study). Along with persistence, compliance is a component of adherence.

In another context, adherence to regulatory and statutory requirements.

Compliance Program Guidance (CPG)

Advice issued by the HHS OIG or FDA to help their staff and the public (including pharmaceutical companies) understand the regulatory rules. Although such guidance is not legally binding, it typically becomes the industry standard of behavior.

compound (or chemical compound)

A distinct substance formed by chemical union of two or more ingredients in definite proportion by weight. In the pharmaceutical context, a compound is not, properly speaking, a medicine or drug until clinical (human) trials have begun.

computational chemistry

The use of computer models to predict the chemical structures/types of compounds that are most likely to have a beneficial effect on a drug target. This discipline is an element of computer-aided drug design.

condition

A term often used synonymously with disease.

consumers

Potential users of pharmaceuticals, their families, and other nonprofessional caregivers. They include people with and without healthcare and/or drug benefits.

continuum of care

Treatment and health management services that encompass all services a consumer might need for a specific illness or across a lifetime, including primary care (e.g., annual checkups), specialty care, hospital treatment, mental healthcare, home healthcare, and long-term care (nursing homes). Continuum of care also implies coordination of healthcare services across all these settings.

contract packaging organization

External provider of packaging services. Some pharmaceutical companies outsource the packaging of their products to a vendor to avoid the high cost of overhead for a packaging facility or the capital expense of building out a facility.

contract pricing

Favorable prices offered by pharmaceutical companies to customers able to drive large prescription volumes. Customers who do not have a special contract with the pharmaceutical company pay a higher standard price. The Federal Supply Service (FSS) is one form of contract pricing. The arrangement may involve discounts off the invoice price, a volume-based reward, or a rebate.

contraindications

Circumstances in which a drug should not be used because the risks clearly outweigh possible benefits. Use of a drug might be contraindicated, for example, because the patient is taking another drug that interacts adversely with it-or because the patient is a member of a special population (children, pregnant women) in whom serious adverse reactions are common.

control group

The subjects in controlled clinical trials who receive a placebo or a drug/dose other than the one being tested. The control group provides a standard against which to measure the efficacy and safety of an investigational drug.

controlled clinical trials

Clinical studies in which one group of participants is given the investigational drug, while another group (the control group) is given either a standard treatment for the disease or a placebo. The FDA requires such trials to establish that a novel drug is sufficiently safe and effective to be marketed.

controlled substances

Drugs classified under the Controlled Substances Act of 1970 as having significant potential for addiction/abuse. There are five controlled-substance categories, known as schedules. Schedule 1 drugs, the most tightly controlled, have high potential for abuse and no recognized medical use. Heroin is one example. The DEA enforces controls on such drugs.

conversion

Switching from one drug to another to treat the same disease or condition.

co-payment

The amount that a consumer who has health coverage contributes toward the cost of health services (including drug prescriptions) that he or she receives. Co-payments are typically flat fees that consumers must pay for each medical expense they incur (e.g., each drug prescription) rather than a percentage of the purchase cost. Many MCOs vary ("tier") drug co-payments to encourage selection of lower-cost or preferred drugs.

For a related concept, see co-insurance.

co-promotion

A form of in-licensing agreement in which a pharmaceutical company purchases a share of the rights to sell and market another company's brand. (That is, Company A and Company B join together to promote a brand.) By contrast, see co-marketing.

Co-promotion rights are typically sold by companies without a sufficiently large in-house sales force to promote their products adequately. Hiring a CSO is an alternative.

cosmeceutical

A cosmetic product claimed to have medicinal or drug-like benefits. Cosmeceutical products are marketed as cosmetics, but reputedly contain biologically active ingredients (e.g., anti-wrinkle skin creams). The cosmetic industry uses the term but the FDA does not recognize this terminology.

counterdetailing

Visits to prescribers by a pharmacists who are paid consultants to a pharmacy benefit management company, an MCO, or other institution. These pharmacists try to counter sales pitches (detailing) for branded products by supplying physicians with unbiased, evidence-based prescribing information to promote the use of generics as a cost-saving measure.

coverage

The type and length of products and services that are covered (or reimburseable), in whole or part, under a healthcare benefits plan.

COX-2 (cyclo-oxygenase-2) inhibitors

A class of non-steroidal anti-inflammatory drug, which works by blocking COX-2-an enzyme whose activity contributes to inflammation.

CPMP (European Committee for Proprietary Medicinal Products)

Within the European Medicines Evaluation Agency (EMEA), the scientific committee that prepares opinions on drugs intended for human use.

CPOs (contract pharmaceutical organizations)

Entities that offer a range of services pharmaceutical companies might want to outsource-such as development, testing, and marketing of products. CPOs are similar to CROs but purportedly offer a more comprehensive range of services.

CPT (Current Procedural Terminology)

A five-digit coding system for services and procedures provided by physicians on an outpatient basis. Developed by the American Medical Association, the system is used for billing to both government and private insurance programs.

CRA (clinical research associate)

An employee of a pharmaceutical company or a CRO or SMO hired by that sponsor, who monitors clinical trial progress at all sites participating in a study. Sometimes called a monitor. The CRA, who usually has a health-care or science background, oversees site initiation, progress, and compliance with the study protocol to protect the scientific integrity of the study and the well-being of study subjects. The role is a combination of administrator, coordinator, consultant, educator, and/or researcher who specializes in clinical trial management.

CRC (clinical research coordinator)

Site administrator for a clinical study, who is based at a single participating medical facility or practice and functions under the supervision of a principal investigator (usually a physician) who is legally accountable for conduct of the study. Also known as a study coordinator, site manager, or research nurse.

CRFs (case report forms)

Records of information collected on each subject during a clinical study (e.g., patient characteristics, medications received, laboratory results, date of visit, adverse events). CRFs are designed by the pharmaceutical sponsor (or CRO) for individual clinical trials.

critical path

In clinical circles, a standardized care regimen, proven to produce the best results for a disease state. In project management, the activities in a project that will take the longest time to complete. Preventing delays in any aspect of the critical path is crucial if activities are to be completed on time.

CRM (customer relationship management)

A system (usually involving specialized software) for tracking and managing all aspects of customer interaction, including marketing, sales and service. Unlike SFA, which is often used synonymously, CRM may not involve the automation of these activities. Account Management and in- and out-bound call centers are components of a CRM system.

CROs (contract research organizations)

A clinical services company working on behalf of pharmaceutical companies. CROs are involved with various steps in the clinical trial and regulatory processes, including study design, trial execution and monitoring, data management and analysis, and regulatory submissions.

crossover trial

A trial in which control groups and test groups switch at the halfway point.

CSOs (contract sales organizations)

"Outside" sales forces that pharmaceutical and biotech companies hire to augment or substitute for an internal sales team.

CTMS (clinical trial management system)

A database that maps study activities and defines the study CRF. It is used to store data generated during the trial and to translate those data stores into reports for the FDA and other regulators.

customer profiling

Collection and analysis of customer information in order to gain insight into their behavior and product preferences.

customer relationship management (CRM)

See CRM.

customer segments

Groups of customers with similar interests in or therapeutic needs for products. Customer segments may be based on age, disease severity, or any number of characteristics. The process of dividing the customer universe into segments is called segmentation.

D

data cleaning (also known as data scrubbing)

In a clinical trial, the process of identifying and resolving any inconsistencies between source documents and case report forms.

database lock

The point after the conclusion of a clinical trial at which all study data have been reviewed and all inconsistencies resolved. After lockdown, the database can no longer be changed. The locked database then undergoes statistical analysis to support NDA submission to the FDA.

DAW (dispense as written)

A notation on a prescription that prohibits the pharmacist from substituting an alternative for the specified product.

DDMAC (Division of Drug Marketing, Advertising and Communications)

The arm of the FDA's CDER charged with ensuring that the information that pharmaceutical companies use to promote pharmaceuticals and biologics (in both marketing materials and product labeling) is truthful and balanced.

Companies do not need to obtain advance approval of their promotional materials but may be required to withdraw them (e.g., TV ads) if DDMAC subsequently determines they are misleading. If a company fails to comply with DDMAC warnings, the penalties can be severe

DEA (Drug Enforcement Administration)

The federal agency that defines and enforces rules for documenting, storing, prescribing, and dispensing controlled substances.

"Dear doctor" or "Dear healthcare professional" letters

Correspondence from the FDA or a pharmaceutical company telling physicians and pharmacists about such issues as adverse effects associated with a particular drug that may be cause for concern and have been identified through post-marketing surveillance.

deciling

Dividing a group of physicians and other potential prescribers for a certain category of drugs into ten segments based on anticipated prescription volume. The highest-volume physicians are in decile 10. (A variant, quintiling, divides physicians into just five segments.)

Deciling allows pharmaceutical companies to place a value on sales calls to each decile, decide which deciles merit in-person detailing, and determine how many sales representatives are required to support the resultant call plan.

deductible

The amount a person with health insurance pays out of pocket for health services before he or she is entitled to any reimbursement from his or her indemnity insurer or managed care organization. Many health plans exempt drug purchases from deductibles, so that a portion of each prescription allowed by that health plan is covered by insurance.

delivery mechanism or delivery method

Often used interchangeably with route of administration, but more specifically refers to the method through which a drug is delivered to the intended organ or receptor site within the body. For example, a drug may be delivered via subcutaneous injection (the route of administration) in formulation that facilitates a controlled release of the active ingredient over time (the delivery mechanism). See also route of administration.

demographics

The characteristics of a population, including sex, age, and family medical history.

depots

Military storage facilities for equipment and supplies. The US Department of Defense and related entities store drugs requisitioned for personnel in depots.

deregistration

The process of removing a drug approved by the FDA (or relevant regulatory entity in other countries) from the market. Deregistration may occur through failure of a pharmaceutical company to re-register a product when the designated registration period has expired or through active intervention by a government to take a product perceived as dangerous off the market.

detail

Sales force presentations to physicians in private practice and their staff, hospital-based medical directors, and retail pharmacists to promote the value of a specific brand or brands. Major pharmaceutical companies have thousands of sales reps "in the field" performing such details.

development

"Umbrella term" for the process of pre-clinical and clinical testing of a candidate compound that culminates, when successful, in approval by the FDA to market a drug.

Also, the function within a pharmaceutical or biotech company that undertakes preclinical and clinical studies.

Development follows discovery, in which the candidate compound is identified.

DHHS (Department of Health and Human Services)

See HHS.

DIA (Drug Information Association)

An organization in which healthcare professionals exchange information on the discovery, development, evaluation, and utilization of drugs. The DIA is noted for the educational programs it provides healthcare professionals.

diagnostics

Branch of medicine dealing with testing to screen a population for illness, to establish or confirm a medical diagnosis in a particular individual, or to determine proper treatment and monitor progress of that treatment.

dialysis

Artificial removal of waste products from the body. It can involve "cleansing" of either the blood (hemodialysis) or the digestive tract (peritoneal dialysis).

diastolic pressure

The lower reading obtained when blood pressure is measured. The diastole is the period when the heart chambers are relaxing and refilling with blood.

Dietary Supplement Health and Education Act of 1994 (DSHEA)

Legislation by the US Congress deregulating the supplement industry, which triggered an explosion in the sale of unproven herbal remedies.

discovery

The search for molecules or compounds that can produce a therapeutic result. Chemical compounds (biologics or synthetics) are investigated in a laboratory setting. When promising candidates have been identified, discovery ends and pre-clinical research begins.

disease

Broadly speaking, any injury, ailment, deformity, disorder, or adverse condition affecting the function of either body or mind. A disease should be capable of diagnosis through specific signs, symptoms, and/or lab results.

disease awareness

Term frequently used by pharmaceutical marketers, who try to increase the market size of a therapeutic area by using direct-to-consumer advertising and physician marketing and educational efforts to "build" awareness of a particular medical condition.

disease pathway

The proteins and protein regulators that cause a particular disease. (The disease may be related to their activity or the absence of normal activity.) By defining a disease pathway, scientists gain insight into genes and proteins that are potential drug targets.

disease management

Programs to diagnose, educate, and/or provide ongoing health status supervision to people with diseases or conditions (usually chronic ones) in order to prevent exacerbation of their health problems and unnecessary consumption of healthcare resources-in other words, for the purposes of controlling costs and maintaining health. These programs are sometimes referred to as health management programs. Initiatives to enhance compliance with the recommended treatment regimen are a common form of disease management program.

dispensing fee

A charge added by pharmacists onto the cost of prescription drugs to reimburse for the application of their professional expertise and the administrative costs associated with filling the prescription.

dispensing pack

Also known as a "carton," this outer casing holds the primary packaging for the drug (e.g., the blister pack). The dispensing pack is the external part of the packaging on which lot and expiration date typically appear.

distribution

During pharmaceutical development, the delivery of the drug to target areas of the body following absorption. On the commercial side, distribution involves the movement of market-ready drugs from manufacturing sites to sites of consumer purchase or use. Wholesalers play a prominent role in this process.

distributors

Companies that transport medical products from manufacturing plants to pharmacies, hospitals, nursing homes, and other provider sites. In the pharmaceutical industry, the major distributors also serve as wholesalers, providing warehouse, packaging, resale and other services to both pharmaceutical companies and providers.

Division of Scientific Investigations

Part of the FDA charged with making on-site inspections to verify that the clinical work cited in an NDA is valid.

DMs (district managers)

Personnel within the sales function who supervise sales representatives. (Structurally, a district is an aggregation of sales force territories.) Their responsibilities include recruiting and hiring sales reps; assessing, coaching, and mentoring them; and overseeing sales analytics that identify primary outreach targets. Sometimes called DSMs (district sales managers).

DMR (direct member reimbursement)

The provision by a payer of reimbursement for a prescription that the member paid for out of pocket.

DNA (deoxyribonucleic acid)

The carrier of genetic information, which provides instructions for creating the hundreds of thousands of human proteins necessary to carry out essential body activities. Genes consist of DNA. The nucleus of every human cell (except blood cells) contains the full DNA complement—that is, the genome—for that person.

DO (Doctor of Osteopathy)

The degree earned by physicians who attend a college of osteopathic medicine. Physicians who graduate from medical school, by contrast, earn an MD. Colleges of osteopathic medicine emphasize a holistic approach to health, focusing on the role of the musculoskeletal system in illness.

DoD

US Department of Defense, which purchases pharmaceuticals for military use. Part of the Federal Markets customer segment.

DoJ

Department of Justice. Federal department that takes an active role in criminal and civil prosecution in such areas as antitrust (often price fixing) and fraud and abuse.

dosage form

The physical medium of the drug (active and inactive ingredients) being delivered. Options include injectable, liquid, dissolved powder, tablet, topical cream, suppository, spray, and transdermal patch.

dose

The amount of a drug administered to a patient or test subject at one time.

dose-ranging study

A clinical trial in which two or more different doses of a drug are tested "head-to-head" to determine which dose works best and is least harmful.

dose-response curve

Relationship between the amount of drug administered and the benefit achieved.

double blind

See blinding.

DPR

See drug price review.

DRG (diagnosis-related group)

An inpatient classification system designed to manage, control, and reduce spending for hospital care. It is based on ICD-9 codes and reflects both primary and secondary diagnoses. These categories are used to define appropriate total reimbursement for a hospital stay. Medicare, for example, provides the same reimbursement amount for every patient coded in a DRG, regardless of differences in actual cost of care. (Medicare pays for hospital outpatient services based on APCs.)

drop ship

A means of distribution in which goods are shipped directly from a wholesaler's (that is, the drug distributor's) warehouse to the customer. The retail "middle man" is left out of the transaction.

drug class

See therapeutic class.

drug delivery

The way in which a drug enters the body, such as orally, through an IV, by inhalation, or by injection. By contrast, dosage form is the physical nature of the drug administered (e.g., tablet, liquid, spray, injectable).

drug design

Approach of discovering new drugs by designing them based on a desired set of chemical and biological responses within the body.

drug discovery

The identification/creation, screening, synthesis, development, and formulation of drugs and the modification of existing agents.

Also, the function within a pharmaceutical company or biotech that undertakes such activities.

drug-drug interactions

The effects that occur when two or more drugs are used simultaneously. Effects may include changes in the drugs' pharmacokinetics, new or more serious side effects, and changes in the drugs' activity.

drug label

See label.

drug maintenance list

A list created by an MCO designating a limited formulary of drugs appropriate for long-term patient use.

drug master file

A submission to the FDA providing detailed confidential information about facilities, processes, or articles used in the manufacturing, processing, packaging, and storing of a drug or drugs.

drug price review (DPR)

A regular update of average wholesale prices (AWPs) from the Blue Book. Health plans use these prices as a basis for defining maximum charges for a drug.

Drug Price Competition and Patent Term Restoration Act of 1984

See Hatch–Waxman Act.

drug product

The finished drug dosage form (such as a tablet, capsule, or cream) resulting from the combination of one or more active pharmaceutical ingredients and (usually) one or more inactive ones. (Placebos, which have no active ingredient, are also considered drug products.)

drugs

The definition provided in the Federal Food, Drug, and Cosmetic Act of 1938 includes "articles intended for use in the diagnosis, cure, mitigation, treatment, or prevention of disease in man or other animals" and "articles (other than food) intended to affect the structure or any function of the body."

The term "drug" is also used by contrast to "biologic" to indicate a product that is chemical in nature.

drug substance

See API.

drug utilization review (DUR)

Retrospective evaluation by MCOs and providers of whether drugs prescribed by physicians were appropriate, given patient condition and formulary guidelines. Based on the results of the reviews, physicians may be required to justify use of expensive or non-formulary drugs before those drugs can be prescribed. See prior authorization.

DTC (direct to consumer)

Marketing materials that are targeted to people who may have a particular disease/condition and/or their families, as opposed to physicians. Typical DTC media include TV and radio ads, magazine and newspaper ads, and consumer-oriented Web sites.

DTP (direct to physician)

Drug marketing targeted to physicians.

dual eligible

A person entitled to receive benefits from both Medicare and Medicaid. The Medicare Prescription Drug Improvement & Modernization Act of 2003 provides that, as of 2006, prescription medications for dual eligibles will be covered exclusively under the Medicare Part D prescription drug program.

DUR

See drug utilization review.

Durham-Humphrey Amendment of 1951

A change in the Federal Food, Drug, and Cosmetic act known as the Prescription Drug Amendment. It established two classes of drugs, prescription and over-the-counter, and vested authority for assigning drugs to each category in the FDA.

Dx

Diagnosis.

E

early adopters

In the pharmaceutical context, physicians, usually key opinion leaders, who are the first to try innovative therapies. They are often targeted by pharmaceutical companies because their usage patterns influence those of other physicians.

ECHO

The acronym for economic, clinical, and humanistic outcomes. Also shorthand for echocardiogram.

edit

A means of altering the way a prescription is dispensed or processed, usually communicated by the payer to the pharmacist at the point of purchase, who then explains the edit to the patient and sometimes the prescriber.

The types of information communicated via an edit include utilization restrictions, pricing and co-payment terms, and formulary non-inclusion.

See point-of-sale edits.

effective dose

Drug dose that causes a defined magnitude of response in a given subject. ED50 is the median dose that causes 50 % of maximal response.

effectiveness

The extent to which a drug produces the intended beneficial effect(s) under the "real world" conditions of typical clinical practice (as opposed to the optimal conditions of the clinical trial environment).

efficacy

The extent to which a drug produces the intended beneficial effect(s) at the dose tested against the designated illness or condition in a clinical trial. Phase 2 clinical trials gauge efficacy, and phase 3 trials confirm it.

EFPIA (European Federation of Pharmaceutical Industries and Associations)

An organization representing the research-based pharmaceutical industry in Europe. It includes national pharmaceutical industry associations and leading pharmaceutical companies.

electronic medical record (EMR)

Computer-based patient record systems.

elimination

The removal of an active drug from the body, either through metabolism or excretion.

EMEA (European Medicines Evaluation Agency)

The entity in the European Union that has drug regulatory responsibilities similar to those of the FDA in the US. Its main responsibility is the protection and promotion of public and animal health, through the evaluation and supervision of medicines for human and veterinary use. Countries in the EU, however, still have the option of maintaining their own drug approval processes.

Emergency Use IND

Emergency Use INDs allow a sponsor to provide an investigational new drug to a treating physician outside of a clinical protocol for use with a patient who has a life-threatening illness. Emergency Use INDs accommodate perhaps a few hundred US patients a year, often HIV patients.

Emergency Use INDs, along with Treatment INDs, are known as Compassionate INDs, but the term "Compassionate" is not in the FDA's IND regulations.

endpoint

The metrics used in clinical trials to judge the effectiveness of a treatment. Endpoint refers to the overall outcome that the study protocol is designed to evaluate. Common endpoints are disease progression, severe toxicity, or death. In some clinical trials, laboratory measurement of some biological indicator of a drug's effectiveness (i.e., a surrogate marker or endpoint) is used in place of longer-term outcome measures. This is particularly common in HIV studies, where CD4 count is used as a surrogate endpoint. See primary endpoint.

enrollee

Narrowly, an individual covered by a health plan who is eligible on his/her own account, not because he/she is a dependent of someone eligible.

Sometimes employed more broadly as a synonym for member, which includes both persons eligible on their own account and their dependents.

enteral

Within or by way of the intestines or the gastrointestinal tract. Enteral feeding involves the provision of nutrition via tubes.

enzyme

A protein that acts as a catalyst, changing the rate at which chemical reactions occur in cells.

EOP (end of phase)

A designation for the conclusion of a stage of clinical trials-e.g., EOP1 is end of phase 1.

e-pharmacies

Web-based entities that allow the ordering and delivery of prescription and over-the-counter drugs over the Internet. They sometimes provide online consultations with healthcare professionals, through which prescriptions are generated.

e-promotions

Promotions and education delivered over the Internet rather than through face-to-face interaction.

epidemiology

A branch of medical science that deals with the incidence, distribution, and control of disease in a population.

episode of care

Healthcare services during a certain uninterrupted period of time, such as a hospital stay.

Sometimes defined as the duration of care of a certain intensity (e.g., ICU care vs. care on a general ward).

EPL (effective patent life)

The portion of a drug's patent life during which it is actually on the market and generating sales.

EPO (exclusive provider organization)

A health plan that provides benefits solely for care obtained from the institutional and professional providers with which it contracts. An EPO may use the same provider network as a PPO, but unlike the PPO will not provide any cover for out-of-network healthcare services. (Exceptions are typically allowed for emergency services and services away from home.)

Generally, EPOs are regulated as insurance companies rather than HMOs.

ERISA (Employee Retirement Income Security Act of 1974) Preemption

A legal doctrine holding that federal law governs the conduct of health plans sponsored by self-insured employers and that, as a result, only federal authorities-not the states-can regulate or challenge the practices of MCOs. In recent years, the courts have limited the scope of ERISA preemption and allowed states to define appropriate MCO practices and/or oppose current practices in court cases related to such issues as utilization control.

ethical drug

A prescription drug (as opposed to an OTC drug) in both the branded and generic forms.

ethical pharmaceutical company

Pharmaceutical companies that develop and sell prescription drugs. Also known as research-based pharmaceutical companies.

etiology

The origin, or cause, of a disease or a patient's symptoms. When the origin is unknown, the disease is called idiopathic.

excipients

The inert substances that are part of almost every drug formulation, in contrast to the active ingredient. They include coloring, flavors, and preservatives. Their purposes include enhancing or maintaining the stability, bioavailability, tolerability, or recognizability of the product.

exclusion criteria

The basis on which potential clinical trial participants are rejected as inappropriate. These criteria are specified in the clinical protocol.

exclusivity

See market exclusivity.

excretion

The elimination of a drug from the body, typically through urine or feces. It is one of the principal means by which the concentration of a drug in the tissues is reduced and drug action is therefore ended.

experience studies

See post-marketing studies.

expression

The manner in which information in a gene is converted to a protein (gene expression)–and information in a protein is converted into activities that may have an impact on health (protein expression).

F

fair balance

The FDA requirement that drug advertisements and promotions equivalently apprise consumers of positive and negative aspects of a medication. For instance, if they extol a drug's efficacy, the advertisements must also provide prominent coverage of side effects and contraindications.

family practitioner (FP)

A physician who provides comprehensive health care to people regardless of age or sex, often placing emphasis on the family unit. Similar to a general practitioner but FPs usually have completed a family practice residency.

Fast Track

An FDA mechanism that expedites review of new drugs to treat a serious or life-threatening disease for which there is an unmet medical need. Under the Fast Track programs, drug sponsors are entitled to early consultation with agency medical reviewers, can rely on surrogate endpoints in clinical trials, and have the option to file certain portions of the NDA in advance of the entire application. Sometimes fast-track drugs are approved based on phase 2 studies. If so, the company must go forward with phase 3 and post-marketing surveillance studies to confirm the benefits of the product.

See Accelerated Approval and Priority Review.

FDA (Food and Drug Administration)

Federal agency, part of the Department of Health and Human Services, that is charged with approving chemical and biologic drugs for marketing in the US and regulating such aspects of marketed drugs as promotion, manufacturing, and adverse events. The FDA monitors all aspects of prescription drugs, while the FTC regulates advertising of OTC products.

FDA-482 form

Notice presented to an investigator, sponsor, or CRO by an FDA inspector announcing the FDA's intent to conduct an inspection.

FD-483 form

Notice issued by an FDA inspector after an inspection describing regulatory violations that were discovered and must be rectified.

FDA-1571 form

Cover sheet for an Investigational New Drug Application submitted to the FDA requesting permission to administer the drug to human subjects.

FDA-1572 form

Signed agreement from a study investigator, acknowledging his/her understanding of the requirements for conducting that study (including the investigator's obligations) and stating that those requirements have been satisfied. Receipt of the FDA 1572 by the sponsor is required prior to shipment of any investigational drugs to that investigator.

FDA Modernization Act of 1997 (FDAMA)

A law that made sweeping changes to the Federal Food, Drug, and Cosmetic Act of 1938. FDAMA was designed to streamline clinical research and make it easier to test and market new drugs. Among other things, FDAMA established a fast-track process for high-priority drugs to treat life-threatening conditions, expanded patient access to investigational drugs, and instituted an extra exclusivity period for products tested in pediatric populations.

Federal Employees Health Benefits Program (FEHBP)

The health benefits program for non-military employees of the federal government (including members of Congress), which is administered by the US Office of Personnel Management. Trend watchers keep track of changes in benefits available from FEHBP, because they often anticipate changes in coverage available to other consumers.

Federal Food, Drug, and Cosmetic Act of 1938 (FDCA)

A statute requiring, for the first time, that manufacturers prove the safety of a drug before marketing it. Among other things, the law states that all print advertisements for drugs must contain a short statement of side effects, contra-indications, and effectiveness, known as the brief summary.

Federal Ceiling Price (FCP)

The maximum price manufacturers can charge for FSS-listed brand name drugs to the four biggest federal purchasers (Department of Defense, VA, Public Health Service, and Coast Guard).

Federal Markets

The federal healthcare procurement system-the largest healthcare system in the US-which includes the Veterans Health Administration (VHA), Public Health Service (PHS), Department of Defense (DoD), and the Indian Health Service. One of the customer segments targeted by Managed Markets account managers.

Federal Register

The "daily awareness" publication of the executive arm of the federal government, which prints calendars of executive meetings and proposed and final rules of bodies such as the FDA.

Federal Trade Commission (FTC)

See FTC.

FFS (fee-for-service) insurance

Traditional insurance, under which providers are paid after the fact for each service actually performed, rather than receiving an advance capitated payment meant to cover all services necessary during a certain time frame. Also known as indemnity insurance. Because fee-for-service systems provide reimbursement for all covered services and products, providers and consumers have little incentive to control utilization.

The vast majority of Medicare enrollees are still in a fee-for-service program.

field sales

Sales reps involved in direct outreach to physicians, other prescribers, and personnel who may exert influence over these prescribers (e.g., office staff).

final dosage form

With respect to a prescription drug product, a finished dosage form, which is approved for administration to a patient without substantial further manufacturing.

first-line therapy

The initial treatment that physicians typically select after diagnosing a specific disease or condition. If it doesn't work, the physician will try a second-line therapy and, if necessary, a third-line therapy.

fiscal intermediary

A private insurance company that contracts with Medicare to carry out the administrative functions of the Medicare program (e.g., making appropriate payments to providers). Fiscal intermediaries handle Medicare Part A and some Medicare Part B bills.

flexible spending account (FSA)

A benefit offered by employers in which a fixed amount of an employee's pre-tax wages are set aside for certain qualified expenses, which include medical costs that standard insurance will not cover (for instance, deductibles, co-payments, and non-covered services). Employees lose any unused dollars in the account at year-end.

formulary

The list of drugs that a managed care organization or hospital favors for use by its enrollees (or that a hospital has approved for use on patients). Use of drugs not on the MCO formulary may be forbidden outright or discouraged through high co-payment requirements. Most formularies encourage use of lower-cost generic drugs and less expensive drugs and select one from a range of similar branded ("me-too") drugs. There are two basic types of formularies-open formularies and closed formularies.

formulary access

See access.

formulation

The substances comprising all active and inert pharmaceutical ingredients, including fillers, colors, and other excipients used to prepare dosage forms.

FSS (Federal Supply Schedule)

The collection of contracts used by federal agencies to purchase supplies and services from outside vendors. FSS prices for pharmaceuticals are negotiated by the VHA and are based on the prices that manufacturers charge their "most-favored" non-federal customers under comparable terms and conditions. (The most-favored customer price may not always be the lowest price in the market.)

fraud and abuse

Most commonly, inflated provider billing to Medicare and other government insurers, such as the various state Medicaid programs. (Privately funded insurance is not the focus of investigation.) In this billing context, fraud involves providers deliberately billing for services that were never rendered, or falsely describing the services actually rendered in order to qualify for higher reimbursement. Abuse occurs when providers unintentionally bill Medicare for items or services they did not provide-for instance, because of poor record keeping.

Although such false billing often receives the greatest publicity, it is not the only form of fraud and abuse. Another important category is some form of kickback (monetary or otherwise) to increase utilization or steer referrals to a certain provider. See antikickback statutes.

Another form of fraud (motivated by a desire among insurers and providers to keep care costs down in a managed care environment) is underutilization of services required to provide quality care to covered patients.

FTC (Federal Trade Commission)

US regulatory agency charged with consumer protection and enforcement of antitrust laws. The FTC regulates the advertising of OTC drugs, with a few exceptions, while the FDA regulates the advertising of prescription drugs. The FTC's antitrust arm monitors the anticompetitive impact of pharmaceutical company mergers, price-fixing efforts, and attempts to keep generic drugs off the market.

fulfillment

The provision of pharmaceuticals to purchasers, typically via some form of pharmacy.

functional genomics

The study (or discovery) of the traits or functions dictated by a given gene sequence. Functional genomics follows upon structural genomics-the identification of the location and "alphabet soup" sequence of a given gene.

G

gatekeeper

Primary care physicians to whom a managed care organization often delegates responsibility for determining whether patients need expensive healthcare services, such as specialist visits, costly lab tests, and inpatient hospitalization. In most MCOs, if the patient bypasses the PCP and goes directly to a specialist without a referral, costs of that specialist visit will not be covered.

GCP (good clinical practice)

Internationally agreed–upon standards for such aspects of clinical trials as study design, data recording, and data analysis. Their goal is to ensure the integrity of data generated from the study and protect the rights of trial subjects.

As part of an IND, a pharmaceutical company must describe the procedures it will follow in clinical trials and explain how its practices will comply with GCP. The FDA issues guidelines on appropriate trial procedures, but they are not legal mandates.

gene delivery

The insertion of genes into selected body cells for such uses as:
- Triggering production of therapeutic agents
- Enhancing susceptibility to a therapeutic agent that has previously been ineffective
- Reducing susceptibility of healthy cells to a therapeutic agent (e.g., to chemotherapy)
- Countering the effects of abnormal genes by inserting normal ones

gene expression

See expression.

gene mapping

The identification of the locations of genes on a chromosome–and the distance between various genes for the purpose of understanding the importance of genes in disease and illness.

general practitioner (GP)

A physician who attends to a variety of medical problems in patients of all ages, rather than focusing on a narrow specialty. Unlike family practitioners, general practitioners have not completed a family practice residency.

generic drugs

Chemically equivalent versions of brand-name ethical drugs for which the patents (and exclusivity rights) have expired. They use the same active ingredients as the brands they mimic, and they must prove bioequivalence with the relevant brand to win FDA approval. They must be identical in dosage form, strength, route of administration, quality, and indications (intended uses). Typically, they must also deliver the same amount of active ingredient in the body over the same time frame.

generic erosion

The loss of sales, profits, and/or market share in the face of generic competition after an ethical brand goes off patent. Manufacturers try to minimize or delay such losses through such means as extending the patent via new indications or isomer drugs or launch of a new product in the same therapeutic area.

generic name

Non-proprietary name of a drug under which it is licensed and identified by the manufacturer. For instance, sildenafil citrate is the generic name for the branded product Viagra. Also, the name of a generic non-branded product (e.g., aspirin).

Generic Pharmaceutical Industry Association (GphA or GPIA)

Organization that represents the generic drug industry and provides lawmakers, government agencies, and regulators with information about the safety and effectiveness of generic medicines.

generic substitution

Replacing the drug specified on a prescription with a generic that contains the same active ingredient as and is bioequivalent to the originally prescribed product. Some MCOs and Medicaid programs mandate generic substitution to reduce drug costs.

genes

The microscopic packets that carry DNA, through which characteristics are passed from one generation to another. Many gene-based tests exist to determine whether a person has a gene mutation associated with a particular disease. Each gene is a segment of double-stranded DNA that holds the recipe for making a specific molecule, usually a protein, and controls the processes related to expression of that protein.

genetic engineering

A form of biotechnology in which genetic material is manipulated to produce desired characteristics. It is also known as recombinant DNA technology. It has been used to manufacture such drugs as insulin, interferon, and growth hormones.

genetic marker

A particular location on the genome in which significant variance occurs. These sites are examined to identify genetic mutations associated with particular diseases.

gene therapy

Insertion of normal or genetically altered genes into cells to treat genetic disorders and chronic diseases. Also known as gene delivery.

genome

All the genes in an organism (e.g., a human, an animal, or a plant). The genome contains one or more chromosomes, depending on the organism's complexity.

genome projects

Research and technology development pursued for the purpose of mapping and sequencing the genome of an organism. The Human Genome Project, a bioinformatics project that has identified the 30,000 genes in human DNA, was one such endeavor.

genomic library

A collection of DNA fragments representing the entire genome of an organism.

genomics

The study of all the genes in an organism and their role in that organism's structure, growth, health, and predisposition to disease.

genotype

All the genes possessed by an individual. Often used more loosely as short-hand for the alleles (variations) at a particular place on the genome.

GFR (glomular filtration rate)

The rate at which the blood is filtered by the kidney. That rate decreases with age and disease.

GLP (Good Laboratory Practice)

Regulations that specify appropriate design, conduct, and reporting of non-clinical laboratory studies-that is, tests on animals. . It does not encompass chemical or microbiological testing of raw materials or products, which are part of GMP. In the US, the FDA has grouped these regulations in the Code of Federal Regulations (21 CFR Part 58).

glidants

A category of excipients commonly known as flow enhancers. They are added to the powders used in pill production to ease movement through the manufacturing equipment. Talc is one example of a glidant.

GMP (Good Manufacturing Practice)

The accepted standards for all aspects of drug manufacturing, including production, packaging, and distribution. It encompasses testing of both raw materials and products. The FDA defines GMP, which it enforces through inspection of manufacturing facilities. The tenets of GMP are enumerated in the Code of Federal Regulations (21 CFR Parts 210 and 211). Both ethical and generics manufacturers must comply.

In non-US markets, the World Health Organization (WHO) also plays a role in defining GMP.

GMP is often referred to as cGMP or current good manufacturing practice to acknowledge that standards evolve and manufacturers must remain current in their practice.

gold standard

In the context of treatment options, the best available option for a disease. Commonly prescribed as a first-line therapy.

In terms of FDA review of an NDA, submission of two independent clinical studies confirming the "substantial effectiveness" of a drug.

GPO (group purchasing organization)

An entity consisting of two or more member hospitals, clinics, or other healthcare entities that band together to obtain favorable purchasing terms for supplies including pharmaceuticals, biologics, and medical-surgical equipment. When members make purchases from suppliers with which the GPO has contracts, they do so at reduced prices.

group health plan

Healthcare coverage purchased by an employer for all its employees or by some other organization, such as an association, on behalf of its members. In contrast to insurance purchased by individuals.

group-model HMO

Structure in which physicians are employed by a group practice that contracts with an HMO and typically see only patients enrolled in that MCO. A variant on the staff-model HMO for use in states that do not permit HMOs to employ physicians.

group purchasing organization

See GPO.

H

haplotype

The combination, within a single person, of various DNA blocks that tend to differ across individuals (that is, contain SNPs). Certain haplotypes seem to be associated with particular diseases. In the future, the efficiency of clinical trials may be enhanced by identifying potential subjects whose haplotypes suggest they might be expected to benefit from or have an adverse reaction to a particular drug.

Hatch-Waxman Act (formally The Drug Price Competition and Patent Term Restoration Act)

A law reflecting a compromise between the interests of generic-drug companies and research-based pharmaceutical companies.

The ANDA (Abbreviated New Drug Application) process it created allowed generic-drug companies to rely on safety and efficacy data for the bioequivalent patented drug in order to obtain FDA approval of their own products. As a result, generics now reach the market much more quickly and their market share has grown enormously.

Research-based pharmaceutical companies, in turn, were given an opportunity for patent extension when a large part of the product's patent life was consumed before the FDA granted marketing approval.

HDMA (Health Distribution Management Association)

A non-profit organization of healthcare and pharmaceutical distributors and manufacturers set up to ensure safe and effective distribution of healthcare products, including pharmaceuticals. It presents the industry position on such issues as bar coding to reduce drug counterfeiting. Formerly known as the National Wholesale Druggists Association (NWDA).

HDL (high-density lipoprotein) cholesterol

The so-called "good" cholesterol that returns to the liver, where it can be eliminated.

healthcare insurers

Companies that assume financial risk for healthcare costs in exchange for receiving coverage premiums from employers, federal agencies, individuals, and other insurance purchasers.

Health Care Financing Administration (HCFA)

See Centers for Medicare and Medicaid Services.

health plan

A managed care benefit package in which financing of healthcare coverage is integrated with aggressive efforts to influence service delivery to the covered population in order to control costs.

Each MCO typically offers a variety of plans to a client with differing levels of restriction on choice and different price points. The least exclusive managed care plans are most costly.

The term "plan" is also used more loosely to refer to an MCO generally, rather than a particular benefits package (among many) offered by that MCO. Less frequently, it is employed to mean any insurer (including fee-for-service ones) whose offerings include utilization controls.

health savings account (HSA)

Funds to which employees and employers can contribute money tax-free, which the employees can draw upon to pay for health services and products, including drug prescriptions. These funds carry over from year to year (unlike funds in FSAs–flexible spending accounts–which are forfeited at year-end if not used). They belong to the employee and are portable if the employee quits or is fired.

HEDIS (Health Employer Data and Information Set)

A set of measures used to evaluate the comparative performance of various health plans, allowing employers who purchase healthcare insurance to make informed choices regarding the best plans to select. HEDIS measures performance based on such characteristics as quality of care, access (that is, ease and speed with which services can be obtained, which is related to such factors as the number of physicians affiliated with the plan), and patient satisfaction.

help-seeking ads

A type of pharmaceutical company ads that are not regulated by the FDA. Help-seeking ads discuss a disease or condition and advise the audience to see a doctor for possible treatments. They need not include any risk information. Because no specific drug product is mentioned or implied, this type of ad is not considered a drug ad.

hemoglobin

The oxygen-carrying pigment of red blood cells. Tests of hemoglobin concentration and for abnormal hemoglobin types identify anemia and other blood diseases.

hepatitis

An inflammation of the liver.

HHS

The US Department of Health and Human Services, of which the FDA and the Centers for Medicare and Medicaid Services are a part. Sometimes abbreviated DHHS.

high prescribers

Physicians and other healthcare professionals who write a large volume of prescriptions in a certain drug class or therapeutic area.

high-throughput screening

Sophisticated technology that allows rapid searches for molecules with desirable characteristics for addressing a particular target. Huge compound libraries can be processed very quickly.

high writers

See high prescribers.

HIPAA (Health Insurance Portability and Accountability Act of 1996)

Also known as the Kennedy-Kassebaum law. A federal law with two main components:

- One pertains to health insurance "portability"-the ability to qualify immediately for comparable health insurance coverage after changing employment.
- The other component, referred to as the Administrative Simplification Section, is designed to ensure an adequate, consistent national standard for controlling the flow of sensitive patient information, particularly through electronic media. Its goal is to protect the security and privacy of health data.

HL-7

Health Level Seven-a technology standard for electronic transfer of healthcare information. HL7 facilitates the transfer of laboratory results, pharmacy data, and other information between different computer systems.

HMOs (health maintenance organizations)

The most restrictive form of MCO, which strives to control healthcare and pharmacy costs by placing sharp limits on the network of covered providers and on utilization of services and products, including drugs. There are two basic models:

- Closed model-Most or all participating physicians are housed in an HMO-owned facility, which typically has an on-site pharmacy. This centralization increases opportunities to manage utilization. Variants include the staff-model HMO and the group-model HMO.
- Independent Practice Association (IPA) model-Independent physicians who have formed a loose affiliation for contracting purposes contract to see HMO patients as part of their private practices. Because IPAs are less cohesive than group practices and work in geographically dispersed offices, opportunities to control utilization through them are more limited than in the closed models.

home health agency

Organization that provides health services to patients in their homes. Services may include skilled nursing, physical therapy, occupational therapy, speech therapy, and assistance with basic activities of living.

home healthcare (HHC)

Health and social support services performed at an individual's home, including part-time nursing care, various types of therapy, assistance with activities of daily living, and meal preparation.

hormones

Chemical substances, usually peptides or steroids, that are formed in one part of the body, travel through the blood, and affect the function of cells elsewhere in the body. Insulin, for example, is a hormone.

hospice

A special care setting for people who are terminally ill and their families. Services include both physical care and counseling.

hospital

An institution whose primary role is the provision of inpatient diagnostic and therapeutic services. Most hospitals also provide some outpatient services, with emergency care being most common.

hospital-based products

In the pharmaceutical context, drugs prescribed and administered on an in-patient basis in a hospital setting rather than prescribed and/or administered in a physician office.

hospitalist

A physician who oversees the care of patients when they are in the hospital. This practitioner will keep the patient's PCP apprised of progress and return the patient to the PCP's supervision at discharge. PCPs avoid the inconvenience of visiting the hospital to check on just one or a few patients. The hospitalist is often employed by the hospital as a means of encouraging PCPs to admit patients to their institution.

HPLC (high-performance liquid chromatography)

A technique for separating a substance into component elements. Its uses include analyses of drug purity.

Human Genome Project

A US-led international effort, begun in 1990 and completed in 2000, to map and sequence the billions of base pairs that make up human DNA. The project was backed and funded by the Department of Energy and the National Institutes of Health.

humanistic outcomes or humanistic studies

One of three broad categories of consequences (outcomes) that are studied in pharmacoeconomic evaluations (the other two being clinical and economic). Humanistic outcomes are the consequences of disease or treatment on patient functional status or quality of life along several dimensions (e.g., satisfaction, general health, physical functioning, social functioning). See pharmacoeconomics and quality of life measures.

I

ICD-9-CM (International Classification of Diseases, Ninth Revision, Clinical Modification)

A coding system for diseases and diagnoses maintained by the World Health Organization. (In the US, the National Center for Health Statistics is entrusted with adapting ICD-9 for domestic use.) It is used to characterize hospital inpatients.

ICD-10 is now used to code and classify mortality data from death certificates, having replaced ICD-9 for this purpose in 1999. When it becomes available, ICD-10-CM, which came out as a draft in June 2003, is planned as the replacement for ICD-9-CM.

ICH (International Council on Harmonization)

A cooperative effort of the FDA and regulatory bodies from Japan and the European Union to reconcile standards so that the same clinical data can be a basis for drug approval in all participating countries. One tangible outcome has been the Good Clinical Practices (ICH-E6) defining international quality assurance standards.

ICU (intensive care unit)

A set of hospital rooms equipped with special equipment, typically used for patients whose condition is unstable and requires close monitoring. Specialized forms of ICU include the NICU (neonatal intensive care unit), SICU (surgical intensive care unit), and CCU (cardiac care unit).

IDN

Integrated delivery network. A single organization, usually built around a hospital or health system, which offers an array of inpatient and outpatient services.

immunology

The study of the body's defense mechanisms against foreign materials that may cause disease or infection.

impurities

Substances that are unintentionally included in a manufactured drug. While such adulterants may not be toxic, the FDA maintains a high purity standard for drugs marketed in the US.

incidence

The number of new cases of a disease, infection, or some other event diagnosed or reported in a specified population during a defined time interval, usually one year. Hypothetical example: "Breast cancer occurs–or recurs–in 1 in 1,000 US women annually." Incidence is often expressed as a rate. Hypothetical example: "In 2004, the incidence of breast cancer in the US was 0.08%." By contrast, see prevalence.

inclusion criteria

The qualifications (such as age, sex, disease severity, general health status) that people must meet to be subjects in a clinical trial.

indemnity insurance

Reimbursement of healthcare providers on a retrospective fee-for-service basis. Indemnity plans do not typically restrict the provider network or have rigorous mechanisms in place to reduce unnecessary product or service utilization and thereby control costs. An insurance system with such control mechanisms, managed care, has largely displaced indemnity plans. Some indemnity programs have tried to adopt similar utilization controls. See managed indemnity.

independent pharmacies

A single retail pharmacy or one that is allied with just a few other local pharmacies. Unlike retail chains, independents do not have a national or regional presence.

IND

See investigational new drug application.

INDA

See investigational new drug application.

Indian Health Service

Agency of the US Public Health Service that provides comprehensive health services to members of federally recognized Indian tribes and their descendants.

indicated

FDA-approved for diagnosis or treatment of a symptom, risk factor, condition, or disease.

indication

A symptom, risk factor, condition, or disease for which the FDA has approved a drug for use. (Sometimes a target population is also specified.) The indication is contained in the product label, also called prescribing information. Drug companies that want to add an indication for an already-marketed drug (to the product label) must file a new application with the FDA. See label or labeling.

infectious diseases

Diseases and disorders that can be passed from person to person or organism to organism, such as hepatitis, tuberculosis, malaria, AIDS, influenza, smallpox, and the common cold. Antibiotics and antiviral agents are frequently used to treat infectious diseases.

informatics

The use of computer technology and statistical analyses to manage information.

See bioinformatics.

informed consent

In clinical trials, voluntary agreement to participate as a subject based upon an adequate understanding of the risks and alternatives. The institutional review board(s) for a trial must approve the consent form used.

infusion

The administration of parenteral drugs (injectables) via an IV.

infusion centers

Sites combining a pharmacy and a clinical services area. Oncology drugs administered intravenously are provided in infusion centers.

injectable

A drug administered via a needle (either syringe or IV infusion). Common modes of injectable administration include subcutaneous, intramuscular, and intravenous.

in-licensing

Typically, acquisition (or sharing) by one pharmaceutical company of the rights to develop and market drugs originated by another pharmaceutical company or biotech company. (Platform technologies are sometimes in-licensed as well.)

inpatient care

Healthcare provided in institutional settings to patients staying for at least 24 hours. Hospitals, skilled nursing facilities, and hospices all provide inpatient services.

in silico

Method by which certain processes or complete scientific experiments are simulated on a computer. Modeling research of this type is frequently conducted as part of pre-clinical research.

institutional providers

Inpatient care settings, such as skilled nursing facilities, hospitals, and long-term care facilities. The corporate leaders of such functions are a target of outreach for Managed Markets account managers. Pharmacists and prescribers within this setting are targets for the sales force.

institutional review boards (IRBs)

Committees of patient advocates, healthcare professionals, and laypersons such as clergy who serve as "watchdogs" to protect the rights and welfare of people participating in clinical trials. They make certain that proposed trials include such safeguards as informed consent to testing and protection of patient privacy. The IRB decides whether a study can begin, oversees its progress, and has the power to stop a study if it seems necessary.

insurance premiums

The payments employers and other purchasers of healthcare coverage make to insurers. Insurers are at financial risk if the actual healthcare costs of the covered population exceed those premiums.

intellectual property (IP)

The rights conferred upon the developer of an original concept or product (e.g., in the pharmaceutical context, a compound). Patents are one form of intellectual property, and pharmaceutical companies with patented products enjoy a period in which no other entity can market exactly the same product.

intensivist

A physician who specializes in oversight of patients admitted to hospital ICUs. A variant on a hospitalist.

intermediate

A material produced during API manufacture that must undergo further purification before it becomes an API.

intermediate care facility

A residential facility that provides health-related care and services to individuals who do not need skilled nursing care, but because of their mental or physical condition require some assistance and supervision.

intern

A physician in training in the first year after graduating from medical school.

internist

A physician who practices internal medicine.

interventions

In a commercial context, actions taken by drug companies, pharmacy providers, PBMs, or other organizations to influence drug selection. Examples include therapeutic substitution, detailing, and educational mailings.

In a healthcare context, intercessions with patients to reverse, avert, or limit the impact of a disease, which may range from behavior modification (diet and exercise) to drug regimens and surgery.

In the context of clinical studies, the treatment or other course of action under investigation.

investigational drug or investigational new drug

A drug being tested on humans for safety and clinical efficacy, which is not yet FDA approved for marketing-or not yet approved for the use, in the dosage form, via the method of administration, or in the combination with other drugs being studied.

Investigational New Drug Application (IND or INDA)

A pharmaceutical company's application to the FDA for permission to test a drug on humans (that is, to conduct clinical trials). The application includes data from pre-clinical testing that support the drug's safety and efficacy, explains the intended use, and describes the clinical protocols for planned human trials. If the FDA does not object within 30 days, clinical testing can begin.

There are three basic types of IND-Commercial, Emergency Use, and Treatment. The latter two forms of IND seek an exemption to give patients with serious or life-threatening diseases/conditions access to promising experimental drugs without being part of a clinical trial.

investigator

A medical professional, usually a physician, who oversees administration of an investigational new drug during a clinical trials He/she is responsible for the conduct and output of that trial. See also principal investigator.

in vitro

Literally translated from Latin, "in glass." In vitro research frequently involves the use of test tubes and other lab implements (e.g., petri dishes) to study or manipulate substances. Such lab work is contrasted with in vivo studies of the effect of substances when administered to people or animals.

in vivo

Internal to the (living) body. Studies of the effects of drugs in humans or animals receiving them are in vivo studies.

IP

See intellectual property.

IPA (independent practice association) model HMO

The most common form of HMO in which individual physicians who have formed a loose affiliation for contracting purposes see HMO patients as part of their private practices. They continue to see "outside" patients as well-both from other HMOs and from other types of payer. IPA-model HMOs rely on providers in their network for medical facilities; they do not own or operate any of their own.

IPAs are considered the HMO model in which HMOs have the least control over physician behavior (including prescription choices). Because IPA-model physicians operate autonomously in different offices and across a relatively broad geography rather than in cohesive groups, it is difficult for HMOs to influence behavior.

IPEC

The International Pharmaceutical Excipients Council, which has independent organizations for the Americas, Europe, and Japan. It is the chief membership organization for excipient producers in the US.

IRB

See institutional review board.

isomer drugs

Compounds with the same molecular formula that differ in structure (link-ages between atoms) or configuration (spatial arrangement of the atoms). An isomer version of an existing product may reduce side effects or have some other beneficial characteristics. Because isomers can be patented separately, they allow pharmaceutical companies with "aging" products to obtain a new period of patent protection.

K

Kefauver rule

A law (the Kefauver-Harris Drug Amendments) passed in 1962 mandating that the FDA receive proof of a drug's efficacy for its intended use before allowing it to be sold in the US. (Prior to this law, only a drug's safety had to be proven.) The law gave the FDA greater regulatory control over clinical trials, instituted more rigorous safety testing requirements, transferred oversight of prescription drug advertising from the FTC to the FDA, and defined good manufacturing practices (GMP) for the pharmaceutical industry.

Kennedy-Kassebaum law

See HIPAA.

key opinion leaders (KOLs)

Scientists (medical researchers), prominent physicians, and leaders from prestigious medical journals, and associations whose opinions on optimal treatment of a specific disease are widely respected. KOLs are able to affect whether a new drug is accepted in the US and globally; their views influence pharmaceutical company customers-payers, prescribing physicians, and consumers.

KOLs

See key opinion leaders.

L

label

Shorthand for the FDA-approved document that specifies each drug's indications and usage, contraindications, adverse reactions, dosage and administration, and other details about the drug. The drug manufacturer furnishes the document for review to the FDA as part of the NDA process. Once the NDA is approved, a pharmaceutical company is prohibited from promoting the product for any purpose (that is, an indication), dosage form, dosage regimen, population, or other parameter other than those approved by the FDA in the product label. The label is also referred to as the package insert, prescribing information, and product information.

Labeling

According to the Federal Food, Drug, and Cosmetic Act, a term broader than "label." Labeling includes "all labels and other written, printed, or graphic matter" that appear on the drug, its contents, or wrappers that accompany the drug. Its scope extends to brochures, booklets, calendars, price lists, exhibits, literature, sound recordings, film strips, file cards, reprints, and letters. Labeling requires full disclosure, which can be satisfied by including the information contained in the approved product label (package insert). The FDA monitors drug labeling for both OTC and prescription drugs.

large molecule

A synonym for biologic compounds, which typically consist of large proteins. Because of their size, large-molecule drugs must often be injected rather than administered orally in a pill or capsule.

latency period

The period after a person is infected with (or otherwise acquires) a disease, but before symptoms of the disease are evident.

launch

The initial entry of a drug into the marketplace–or the entry of an established drug into a new market for which the manufacturer has received an additional indication.

LCA (least costly alternative)

The price assigned by Medicare to a drug it considers worthy of reimbursement, but not at a price premium to competitors in the same drug class. To "LCA" a drug, Medicare regulators determine the equivalent dose for another drug in the same class, then enforce the least expensive drug's reimbursement rate per dose. In the absence of an LCA, a drug is typically reimbursed by Medicare based on AWP (average wholesale price).

LDL (low-density lipoprotein) cholesterol

The "bad" cholesterol that is carried into the blood and is the main cause of harmful fatty buildup in arteries. High LDL levels increase the risk of heart disease.

lead identification

The process of finding compounds or molecules that will have a beneficial impact on a disease-related target.

lead compound

A compound that shows promise as a drug therapy because of its biological effects against a selected disease-related target. The best of related lead compounds becomes a candidate compound.

lead optimization

The effort to maximize the efficacy and minimize the side effects of a lead compound.

lead series

A group of compounds that vary structurally in small ways. They are studied to learn the effect of structure on drug activity, which facilitates compound optimization. See structure-activity relationships.

legend drug

A drug that can only be obtained with a prescription. The term comes from the legend (or label) on each prescription, which states, "Federal law prohibits dispensing without a prescription."

LESI (Licensing Executives Society International))

An association of national and regional societies, each composed of men and women who have an interest in the transfer of technology or licensing of intellectual property rights. An organization that includes business development managers within the pharmaceutical industry.

lesion

Almost any damage to tissue, including a tumor, scarring (external or, for instance, on the lungs), a pimple, and a stomach ulcer.

licensing

A function performed by the Business Development group within a pharmaceutical company, which involves buying and selling rights to compounds, drugs, research technologies, or other assets. See in-licensing and out-licensing.

life cycle

The series of stages that a branded drug passes through, from discovery to patent and clinical trials to launch and market maturity and on to patent expiration and the entry of generic competition.

life cycle management

Adjustments to product strategy to maximize market share and revenues in various stages of a brand's patent life (e.g., launch, entry of new competition, imminent patent expiration). Contingency planning for a compound's commercial future begins during discovery.

lifestyle drugs

Term used for drugs that enhance quality of life, but are not considered medically necessary. Erectile dysfunction, skin care, and hair replacement therapies are key examples.

ligands

Drugs that exert their effect by triggering or blocking receptor action.

line extensions

New formulations and new means of delivering an already-marketed chemical entity, rather than an NCE. Examples include new strengths, dosage forms, or combinations of drugs. Line extensions undergo clinical testing and often demonstrate substantial benefits in terms of efficacy, ease of administration, and patient compliance. A substantial portion of pharmaceutical industry research and revenue comes from line extensions.

LMRP (local medical review policy)

The effort of a Medicare fiscal intermediary to decide whether to cover a new outpatient drug for which Medicare has defined no overarching national coverage policy. See NCD (national coverage determination).

long-term care (LTC)

Custodial and non-custodial care provided to people with disabilities or chronic/long-term health needs. Forms of LTC include skilled nursing, eldercare, and assisted living facilities (ALFs).

long-term care hospital

Under Medicare rules, a hospital with an ALOS of 25 or more days. Such institutions provide extended medical and rehabilitative treatment for patients with complex, acute health problems or multisystem failure. Often, these patients are medically unstable and require frequent treatment interventions and/or rehabilitation sessions.

long-term care pharmacy providers (LTCPP)

Entities licensed to dispense to residents of long-term care facilities.

LOS (length of stay)

Number of days a patient spends in a hospital or other healthcare facility-or in a particular unit of that institution (e.g., the ICU).

LPN (licensed practical nurse)

A nurse whose training and responsibilities are less extensive than that of a registered nurse (RN). LPNs usually have a year of post–high school training and state certification. Working under an RN's or physician's supervision, an LPN provides care such as administering treatments, bathing patients, changing dressings, and checking temperature and blood pressure.

M

mail-order pharmacy

A popular method of dispensing medication for chronic conditions or lifestyle drugs directly to patients. Prescriptions are typically mailed to the pharmacy by patients or faxed to the pharmacy by a physician.

major statement

The most important risks associated with a drug, which the FDA mandates must be displayed prominently (or stated) in TV and radio ads promoting that drug.

managed behavioral healthcare organization (MBHO)

An MCO that specializes in the management, administration, and/or provision of mental health benefits. Like other MCOs, they employ utilization controls to keep care costs down.

managed care

A largely but not exclusively private health insurance sector made up of MCOs, which emphasizes controls to ensure cost-effective care. Typically, a central administrator is paid a fixed amount of money per member per month and is at risk for losses if the actual cost exceeds that payment. That administrator uses a variety of devices to discourage healthcare providers (physicians and hospitals) from using unnecessarily costly therapeutic products and services.

managed care organizations (MCOs)

Health insurers that keep down the cost of care by controlling overall utilization and, particularly, access to expensive health resources (specialists, expensive drugs, and so on). PPOs and HMOs are two types of MCO.

managed fee-for-service plans

Health plans in which the insurer pays healthcare providers (e.g., physicians and hospitals) retrospectively based on actual services rendered, but incorporates some utilization controls as well, such as prospective length-of-stay approval for inpatient admissions, second opinions for surgery, and claims audits.

managed indemnity

See managed fee-for-service plans.

Managed Markets (function)

The people within a pharmaceutical company who are charged with developing a strategy for winning favorable payer coverage of company brands. "Managed Care" is sometimes used as a synonym, as is "Managed Markets Marketing." Managed Markets strategy is carried out by account managers who call on payers.

Managed Markets (segments)

The discrete customer groups targeted by the Managed Markets function-Trade (wholesalers and the corporate headquarters personnel of retail pharmacies), Federal Markets (the VHA, DoD, and others), MCOs, Long-Term Care, and Medicaid/Medicare.

mandatory generic program

A health plan requiring that members use generic drug products when available. Members who choose to use the brand product rather than the generic will bear a greater share of the cost of the medication-and in some cases, the entire cost.

manufacturing

All the steps involved in making a finished drug product ready for marketing, which include not only production of the active ingredient in a formulation, but also packaging, labeling, and storage.

market-based pricing

The practice of employing different price schemes for the same product in different countries or regions of the world.

market basket

A product's therapeutic classification and its important competitors. Marketing and selling strategies are designed to differentiate the product from others in the market basket, and market share performance is measured against other products in the market basket.

market exclusivity

A grant from the FDA of exclusive marketing rights for an FDA-approved drug-that is, protection from FDA approval of a generic version. The protection extends from the point of NDA or ANDA approval:

- 7 years for orphan drugs
- 5 years for an NCE (new chemical entity)
- 3 years for improvements on existing drugs (during which the original version of the drug cannot be challenged by a generic either)
- 6 months added to applicable exclusivity/patent period if a drug is tested for use in children
- 180 days of exclusivity to generics companies that launch successful patent challenges

Exclusivity is separate from rights conferred under a patent from the USPTO. The FDA can grant exclusivity rights, for instance, on a product that is not yet patented or one for which the patent has expired. The exclusivity period, however, cannot be added on to the patent life.

market expansion studies

Phase 4 studies conducted for the purpose of promoting newly FDA-approved uses (indications) of a drug among a large group of target physicians and patients.

marketing

See Brand Management and Marketing.

marketing manager

Within Brand Management, the person responsible for a specific communications channel (e.g., TV or Web) or customer segment for a brand or brand indication. Often recruited from Market Research, Medical Communications, or Sales.

Market Research

A function within a pharmaceutical company (or an outside vendor) that performs primary research (interviews, focus groups, surveys), secondary research, and analyses. Market Research supports Brand Management, Managed Markets, and Business Development planning.

mass spectrometry

A technique for identifying substances present in a sample and the purity of a substance or compound (the extent to which unintended substances, or adulterants, have crept in). The machine employed is known as a mass spectrometer.

Maximum Allowable Cost (MAC)

A cost management program that sets upper limits on the unit price that will be paid for equivalent generic drugs available from different manufacturers. Medicaid and many private payers have MAC lists that they use to control the costs of generics.

Also, in the context of AIDS or HIV, mycobacterium avium complex.

MDC (major diagnostic category)

A classification system that represents a group of similar diagnosis-related groups (DRGs). Each MDC typically involves a single organ system of the body.

mechanism of action (MOA)

The means by which the active ingredient in a drug exerts its effect (therapeutic or toxic) on the body. Or, the manner in which a disease or condition is produced.

Scientists attempt to identify the mechanism of action through preclinical research, but in a surprising number of cases, the precise mechanism of action of a drug remains unknown, although clinical studies demonstrate that the drug is in fact an effective therapy.

Medicaid

The health insurance program for the poor and disabled administered by each state and funded by money from that state and from the federal government. In contrast to Medicare, which is insurance for persons aged 65 or older and certain disabled persons, Medicaid is for people under age 65 who are below the poverty level and, therefore, cannot afford private health insurance. Medicaid plans vary from state to state, although the federal government mandates that each program include certain basic elements. Medicaid plans include a broad-based outpatient drug benefit.

Medicaid Prescription Drug Rebate Program

A pricing system created by the Omnibus Budget Reconciliation Act (OBRA) of 1990, designed to leverage Medicaid's purchasing power by requiring the same kind of volume discounts afforded to other large purchasers of prescription drugs. Pharmaceutical companies that choose to participate in the rebate program obtain Medicaid coverage for most FDA-approved drugs. States, in turn, receive rebate dollars.

Medicaid price

A discount off average wholesale price (AWP). For branded drugs, the required rebate is the greater of 15.1% of AMP or AMP minus the best price offered another purchaser.

Medicaid Prudent Pharmaceutical Purchasing Act (MPPPA)

Legislation, passed as part of the Omnibus Budget Reconciliation Act of 1990, which mandates that Medicaid receive the best price offered to any institutional purchaser. Drug companies provide rebates to Medicaid to the difference between that discounted price and the price at which the drug was sold.

Medical Affairs (function)

Clinical development specialists (often physicians, PharmDs, CRAs) who help the commercial side of the company conduct clinically oriented phase 4 studies after product launch. They also act as a general clinical "resource" to answer sales representatives' questions, field product inquiries from physicians, and interact with key opinion leaders.

Medical Communications (function)

A group within a pharmaceutical company responsible for various aspects of communicating medical information to customers, payers, and regulators. Responsibilities within this group may include product launch support, clinical monographs, drug information services, medical writing, slide kits, claims substantiation documentation, managed care dossiers, speaker programs, advisory boards, sales ads, and advocacy programs to educate and encourage support for a product. Many of these functions are contracted out to medical communication companies.

medical communications companies

Vendors hired by pharmaceutical companies to create and implement the various functions of Medical Communications.

medical devices

Like drugs, medical devices are used in diagnosis, treatment, or prevention of diseases or conditions-or to affect the structure or function of the body. Unlike drugs, they produce their principal benefit in some way other than chemical action in or on the body. The many varieties include laser systems for vision correction, x-ray machines, crutches and wheelchairs, and materials used or inserted during surgery such as pacemakers and stents. In the pharmaceutical context, equipment used to administer drugs such as inhalers for asthma products and epinephrine autoinjectors for severe allergic reactions are medical devices.

medical protocols

Step-by-step guidelines that are supposed to produce the optimal outcome in treatment of a disease or condition. They are typically based on accumulated medical research about clinical outcomes under different therapeutic regimens.

See clinical protocols.

medical reviewers

Personnel (usually physicians and often called medical officers) employed by the FDA who approve the clinical portions of applications such as INDs (safety of the protocol) and NDA (validity of test results). Also known as clinical reviewers.

medical science liaisons (MSLs)

Healthcare professionals (often within Medical Affairs) in a pharmaceutical company who work closely with key opinion leaders in the relevant therapeutic area to share preliminary findings from ongoing clinical trials, information about planned phase 4 studies, and data on off-label drug use with interested prescribers, as allowed under guidelines set forth by the FDA. To avoid any taint of sales bias in presenting such product information, Medical Affairs does not report to Sales. They are a resource to whom prescribers turn with clinical and scientific questions.

medical staff

Professional medical personnel who provide care to patients in an organized facility, institution, or agency.

Medicare

Federally funded health insurance for persons age 65 or older, as well as younger persons with certain disabling conditions, such as end-stage renal disease. It includes both Part A (free hospital insurance) and Part B (optional medical insurance for which beneficiaries must pay a monthly premium, which provides coverage for physician services provided outside the hospital, durable medical equipment, and selective other therapies).

Medicare and Medicaid Patient Protection Act of 1987

The federal "antikickback statute" forbidding monetary and non-monetary rewards to physicians and other healthcare personnel to encourage them to use or recommend that patients use particular products or service providers. See antikickback laws.

Medicare carrier

A private company that contracts with Medicare to pay most Part B bills. A carrier is the Medicare Part B equivalent of a fiscal intermediary (which handles Medicare Part A bills and a few types of Part B bills).

Medicare drug discount card

A program implemented in 2004 to provide Medicare beneficiaries with an opportunity to reduce the costs of prescription drug purchases prior to the implementation of a broader Medicare outpatient prescription benefit to begin in January 2006. See Medicare prescription drug benefit

Medicare exclusions

Items or services that Medicare does not cover, such as long-term care and custodial care in a skilled nursing facility or private home. Traditionally, these exclusions also included most drugs that are self-administered on an outpatient basis, but that situation is changing. See Medicare Prescription Drug Improvement & Modernization Act.

Exclusions are also known as Medicare gaps.

Medicare Part A

Known as the hospital insurance component of Medicare. Part A pays for inpatient hospital stays, (relatively brief) care in skilled nursing facilities, some home healthcare, and hospice care.

Medicare Part B

Known as the medical insurance component of Medicare. Part B helps pay for physician services provided outside hospitals (and for drugs administered as part of those services), lab and radiology services, ambulance service, outpatient hospital care, durable medical equipment; some other medical services that Part A does not cover, such as physical and occupational therapy and limited home healthcare.

Traditionally, Part B drug coverage has been limited to a small number of products (typically very expensive products). Reimbursed pharmaceuticals and biologics included blood transfusions, immunosuppressive drugs (for transplant patients), and oral anti-cancer drugs. A broader drug benefit has now been established. See Medicare Prescription Drug Improvement & Modernization Act.

Medicare Part B, unlike Part A, is not free and, therefore, some people opt not to carry this coverage.

Medicare Prescription Drug Improvement & Modernization Act (MMA)

Legislation passed by Congress in 2003 that established coverage for a broader array of outpatient prescription drugs used by Medicare patients. The MMA has several key provisions. The transitional Medicare-endorsed drug discount program, which provides voluntary prescription drug benefits to certain eligible beneficiaries, will terminate at the end of December 2005 as the Medicare Part D prescription drug benefit goes into effect in January 2006, at which time Medicare beneficiaries will receive outpatient prescription drug coverage. This voluntary drug benefit will be delivered through private risk-bearing entities under contract with the Department of Health and Human Services.

The MMA also includes changes to the reimbursement approach for drugs covered under Part B-moving from a system that reimbursed for products based on average wholesale price (AWP) to one that reimburses on average sales price (ASP) plus 6%. Also in 2006, Medicare/Medicaid dual-eligible individuals will begin receiving their prescription drug benefits through Medicare Part D rather than state Medicaid programs.

Medicare+Choice

Spoken as "Medicare plus Choice." A managed care option for Medicare enrollees that provides some supplemental benefits not available under standard fee-for-service Medicare. One major selling point, now moot due to changes in the basic Medicare program, was the inclusion of an outpatient drug benefit.

Medicare prescription drug benefit (Medicare Part D)

New prescription drug benefit covered under the Medicare Prescription Drug Improvement & Modernization Act. The Part D drug benefit, which goes into effect in January 2006, will be provided by private health plans and is a voluntary program for Medicare beneficiaries (except for dual-eligible individuals).

All Medicare beneficiaries may obtain prescription drug coverage by either: remaining in the traditional Medicare fee-for-service program and adding a stand-alone prescription drug benefit provided by a PBM or MCO or selecting one of several alternative programs provided through private insurers, PPOs, HMOs, or PBMs. Beneficiary deductibles and co-pays will differ by federal poverty level. See Medicare Prescription Drug Improvement & Modernization Act.

medicinal chemistry

The identification, synthesis, and development of new chemical entities suitable for therapeutic use. It requires knowledge of (among other things) chemistry, biochemistry, immunology, pharmacology, and computer-based research technologies.

medicinal chemistry laboratories

Entities hired by pharmaceutical companies to transform a drug in development into a usable form (e.g., create a formulation that stabilizes the active ingredient or turn an injectable into a pill).

medicine

The science of diagnosing, treating, or preventing disease and other damage to the body or mind. The term is also used to refer to any substance used to treat or prevent disease or other damage to the body or mind.

Medigap

Formally known as the Medicare supplemental health insurance policy. Medigap insurance is sold by private insurance companies to Medicare beneficiaries to cover specific expenses either not covered or not fully reimbursed by Medicare.

M/E

Meetings and events, a component of promotional spending that is primarily directed to physicians. Its scope includes conferences and continuing medical education programs.

MedWatch

Part of the FDA's post-marketing surveillance system, established in 1993 to make it easier for healthcare professionals and consumers to report health problems and adverse events related to prescription and OTC drugs, biologics, and medical devices. If a causal relationship is found between adverse events reported by these groups and a particular drug, FDA officials decide whether some form of public notification , or even withdrawal of the drug from the market, is needed.

members

Participants in a health plan (enrollees or eligible dependents).

metabolic pathway

A chain of enzyme reactions occurring in living cells that transforms one compound into another one (either breaking down a large compound or building (synthesizing) a larger one. Researchers are studying the relationship between specific variants of genes and proteins and specific metabolic pathways in order to gain insight into disease causation.

metabolism

A biological process that changes chemical structures and the properties of chemical compounds. Most drug metabolism in the human body occurs through the action of enzymes in the liver, which breaks down potentially toxic substances. Metabolized drugs become more water soluble and therefore more easily eliminated from the body.

People with damaged livers have trouble metabolizing drugs and, thus, are at higher risk of toxic effects. Drug metabolism can also be affected by factors like genetics, age, sex, foods ingested, and environmental hazards, such as smoking and pesticides.

metabolites

Chemical compounds produced in the body as a result of metabolic reactions.

method of administration

See route of administration.

"me too" drug

A new patented brand that has a different active ingredient than an already-marketed ethical drug but uses the same therapeutic mechanism of action and therefore competes with it directly. The two drugs are typically very similar in structure and differ only slightly in characteristics such as safety, efficacy, and tolerability.

milestone payments

Payments that "come due" only upon achievement of some specific goal (e.g., entry of a compound into phase 3 trials or realization of a certain level of sales revenues from a product). If the milestone is never achieved, no payment is made.

Ministry of Health, Labor, and Welfare (MLHW)

One of the agencies responsible for drug evaluation in Japan. The Pharmaceutical and Medical Safety Bureau within MLHW oversees the safety and efficacy of drugs, cosmetics, and medical devices.

mirrored territories

Territories in which two or more reps promote the same products to the same prescribers. The goal is to optimize the number of sales details to target physicians, given the distinctly limited number of times a physician is likely to be willing to see any one sales rep.

misbranding

Labeling or advertising that is misleading.

mixed-model HMOs

HMOs that represent a hybrid of the standard models. A staff- or group-model HMO that expanded its provider network by negotiating with an IPA would be a mixed model.

MMA (Medical Marketing Association)

A non-profit organization whose membership consists of marketing professionals from the pharmaceutical, medical device, and diagnostic industries.

molecular modeling

The process of generating a visual representation of the 3-D structure of a biologic molecule (for instance, a drug target), in order to guide drug discovery efforts. Molecular modeling speeds the definition of structure–activity relationships and the design of new (drug) molecules that will be effective on the target.

molecule

A group of atoms held together by chemical forces. The smallest unit of a compound that possesses all characteristics of that compound.

monitor

A person employed by a clinical trial sponsor or CRO who reviews study records for compliance with the trial protocol. CRA is a synonym.

monoclonal antibodies (MAbs or MOAbs)

Laboratory-produced proteins of unusual specificity that can replicate indefinitely and "lock in" on just one antigen. Their applications to date are primarily in cancer. This type of therapy is an effective means of helping patients with compromised immune systems fight tumors.

monograph

See product monograph.

monotherapy

The sole therapy employed, as opposed to combination therapy.

morbidity

A disease or the incidence of disease within a population. Also, adverse effects caused by a treatment.

mRNA (messenger RNA)

The template for creation of proteins (that is, protein synthesis) generated by DNA. In other words, the "messenger" that takes DNA information and converts it to protein production.

MSA (medical services account)

A benefits program in which consumers are allocated a lump sum of money for prospective medical expenses to spend as they see fit.

MSLs

See medical science liaisons.

multispecialty group

Physicians from a variety of specialties who work together in a group practice.

multisource products

Pharmaceutically equivalent products (from multiple companies) that may or may not be therapeutically equivalent. Multisource pharmaceutical products that are therapeutically equivalent are considered interchangeable.

N

NACDS (National Association of Chain Drug Stores)

The largest US pharmacy association. The chain community pharmacy industry includes traditional chain drug stores, supermarket pharmacies, and mass-merchant pharmacies.

naïve patients

People with a condition or disease who haven't previously been on a particular type of treatment or in some cases any treatment. Patients may be treatment-naïve, drug-naïve, or naïve to a particular drug class. Naïve patients are desirable in studies because their bodies have not built up a resistance to a drug that might otherwise be effective.

NAM (national account manager)

An account manager in a pharmaceutical company who organizes managed markets outreach on a national rather than a regional basis.

narrow therapeutic index (NTI)

A very limited dosing range in which a drug is both effective and not prohibitively toxic. Drugs with an NTI are called dose sensitive.

National Center for Health Statistics (NCHS)

A division of the US Department of Health and Human Services and one of the Centers for Disease Control and Prevention (CDC). The principal source of health statistics for the nation, NCHS gathers data on illness and disability, as well as on the use and availability of health services.

National Formulary

An official publication, issued first by the American Pharmaceutical Association and now yearly by the United States Pharmacopeial Convention as part of the USP-NF, which describes standards for excipients, botanicals, and other similar products.

Also, the list of approved drugs established by such payers as the Department of Veterans Affairs.

National Institutes of Health (NIH)

The federally funded medical research organization based in Bethesda, MD. It spends billions of dollars each year on research to enhance understanding of disease. The information NIH has produced regarding mechanisms of disease has contributed to drug discovery efforts by pharmaceutical companies.

NCE

See new chemical entity.

National Community Pharmacists Association (NCPA)

An organization that represents the owners, managers, and employees of independent community pharmacies in the US.

NCD (national coverage determination)

A ruling by Medicare at the national level regarding whether an outpatient drug will be covered. Such a national ruling supersedes any contrary coverage determinations made by local carriers. See LMRP. Manufacturers may request an NCD in hopes of obtaining a favorable ruling that means their product will be reimbursed by Medicare carriers in all localities.

NCPDP (National Council for Prescription Drug Programs, Inc.)

A not-for-profit standards-development organization for the pharmacy services industry. It developed the official standard for e-transmission of pharmacy claims under HIPAA.

NCQA (National Committee for Quality Assurance)

A non-profit organization that accredits and measures the quality of care in managed care health plans.

NDA (New Drug Application)

A lengthy document requesting permission from CDER to market a new drug (usually a non-biologic) that has undergone phase 1, 2, and usually phase 3 clinical trials. The FDA needs to determine, based on the evidence submitted, whether the drug is safe and effective for its proposed use(s) and whether its benefits outweigh its risks. The FDA also scrutinizes such aspects of the NDA as the description of proposed manufacturing processes and the accuracy of its proposed labeling.

Once the FDA approves the NDA, a pharmaceutical company may launch and promote the product.

NDC (national drug code)

A unique FDA-assigned code used to track a pharmaceutical product throughout the supply chain. It appears on manufacturer price lists, the package insert, and the prescription label prepared in a pharmacy. The coding system is a "common language" for manufacturers, wholesalers, pharmacies, clinics, and any other organizations that handle the product. It is roughly the equivalent, for drugs, of the universal product code (UPC) on other products.

NDC block or lockout

An MCO directive forbidding a pharmacist to dispense a product (identified by its national drug code) to its members. Lockouts are a means of excluding certain products in a generally open formulary.

net loss ratio

An insurer's total liability (from beneficiary claims) and other expenses, divided by the premiums it has been paid.

network

A group of physicians, hospitals, pharmacies, and other healthcare providers that agrees to restrictions on fees and compliance with usage controls in exchange for inclusion in a managed care health plan.

The point of a network is to create a small circle of providers that the MCO can manage to control utilization of health resources. A "closed" network is one in which beneficiaries cannot use out-of-network providers (if they want the MCO to pay for care); an "open" network allows beneficiaries to use out-of-network providers, but makes them pay a higher share of care costs.

network-model HMO

A type of open-model HMO in which the MCO contracts with multiple (typically large) physician groups to care for their patients, while the physician groups are free to see patients outside of the MCO membership. Because groups are typically paid communally and on a capitated basis, they have a strong shared incentive to control unnecessary healthcare expenditures. The HMO's ability to influence utilization practices is considered greater than under the IPA model–but less than under a group or staff model.

new chemical entities (NCEs)

Defined in the Hatch–Waxman Act as a chemical compound not previously approved for use in humans by CDER. The term excludes diagnostic agents, vaccines, and other biologic compounds not approved by CDER, as well as new salts, esters, and dosage forms of previously approved compounds. NCEs enjoy a longer period of exclusivity (five year) than other branded drugs.

Often used interchangeably with new molecular entities, although new molecular entities would also encompass biologics in addition to chemical compounds.

new molecular entities (NMEs)

See new chemical entities.

NOC (Notice of Compliance)

Roughly the Canadian equivalent of FDA approval of an NDA, which allows a product to be sold in Canada. The issuance of an NOC indicates that a drug meets the required Health Canada standards for use in humans or animals.

non-approvable letter

An FDA response to an NDA listing major deficiencies that will preclude approval if not corrected.

nonparticipating provider

A physician (or other healthcare professional or institution) who has not contracted with a particular health plan to provide care. If the provider nonetheless agrees to provide services, it will be an "out–of–network" provider.

nonpreferred drug

A disfavored alternative to a preferred drug, which may not be on the payer formulary at all. It usually carries a high co-payment to discourage use and may also involve restrictions such as a prior authorization requirement.

nosocomial infection

An infection acquired in the hospital. For instance, nosocomial pneumonia is synonymous with hospital-acquired pneumonia.

notice of violation (NOV)

The most common type of regulatory action by the FDA, citing a violation of applicable laws or regulations.

NSAIDs (non-steroidal anti-inflammatory drugs)

Pronounced en-seds. A category of drugs used to treat pain and inflammation in a variety of conditions. As their name indicates, they do not contain cortisone or other steroid drugs. The most commonly used NSAIDs are aspirin, ibuprofen, and naproxen. .

nuclear medicine

A medical specialty involving the use of very small amounts of radioactive materials or radiopharmaceuticals to create body images in order to diagnose, manage, treat, and prevent disease. Nuclear medicine imaging reveals organ function and structure, in contrast to diagnostic radiology (e.g., x-raying), which merely provides a snapshot of anatomy. Today, every major organ system can be examined via nuclear medicine.

nucleic acid

The molecules of which DNA-deoxyribonucleic acid-is composed.

nucleotides

The four "building blocks" of which all DNA is made. They are generally represented by the letters A, C, G, and T. See base pairs.

nurse's aide

An individual who provides basic nursing care under the supervision of a registered nurse or an licensed practical nurse; also called nurse's assistant, nursing attendant, healthcare assistant, or orderly.

nurse practitioner

An RN with two or more years of advanced training (including coursework in clinical pharmacology) who has passed a special exam. Such nurses can take on some of a doctor's normal functions (especially in a primary care setting) such as physical exams, diagnostic testing, and the development of treatment plans. In some states, nurse practitioners can write prescriptions.

nursing home

Typically a layman's term rather than one employed by healthcare professionals, signifying an entity that custodial nursing and/or personal care to the aged, infirm, or chronically ill. See SNF.

nutraceuticals

A popular (rather than a regulatory) term for products that combine traditional food ingredients with active ingredients alleged to provide health benefits that are not purely nutritional. They include vitamins and other nutritional supplements and so-called "functional foods" like bran.

NWDA (National Wholesale Druggists Association)

Former name of the HDMA (Health Distribution Management Association). See HDMA.

O

observational studies

Studies in which the investigators do not manipulate the use of an intervention (e.g., patients are not randomly assigned to a treatment or control group), but only observe patients who are (or are not) exposed to the intervention, and interpret the outcomes. Observational studies are considered less rigorous, and their results less reliable, than randomized, controlled studies.

OBRA (Omnibus Budget Reconciliation Act) of 1990

A federal law specifying that pharmaceutical companies that want drugs taken on an outpatient basis to be covered by Medicaid must provide best price rebates to Medicaid programs. For brand-name drugs, the minimum rebate is 15.1% of the average manufacturer price (AMP).

office-based products

Products typically prescribed in a physician's office that may be dispensed in that setting (e.g., vaccines) or through a retail pharmacy.

off-label drug use

Use of a drug for a purpose (that is, an indication), in a dosage form, or dosage regimen, population, or other parameter other than those approved by the FDA as stated on the product label (package insert). Physicians are free to experiment with off-label uses, but pharmaceutical companies cannot promote such uses to prescribers or consumers. The ways pharmaceutical companies can share information about off-label uses with physicians are sharply circumscribed by the FDA.

off-patent

A term for non-generic drugs whose patents have expired, as in "Taxol went off-patent in 2001."

OIG (Office of Inspector General)

The group within a US regulatory agency responsible for ensuring the integrity of programs administered by that agency. The OIG of greatest interest to the pharmaceutical industry is in HHS. It combines its enforcement role with an advisory one; among other things, the HHS OIG has issued guidance on compliance with FDA rules about product promotion to physicians.

oncology

Study and treatment of cancer.

online adjudication

Electronic validation of a drug benefit claim at the location where a prescription is dispensed-for example, the pharmacy. The purpose is to determine potential coverage problems before the drug is dispensed to the patient.

online pharmacies

Entities that sell drugs-OTC and sometimes prescription as well-through the Internet.

open formulary

The provision of reimbursement for drugs that are not on an MCO or PBM formulary (list of preferred products). While the payer favors use of formulary drugs, it will offer coverage for nonformulary products as well, but will usually require a higher co-payment.

open-label study

A clinical trial in which study subjects and researchers both know the treatment and dose being administered to that subject. Usually in open-label studies all patients receive the same medication-there is no control group.

open-panel HMO

An HMO that contracts with physicians in private practice to see HMO enrollees as well. Unlike a closed-panel HMO, open panels do not require participating physicians to see only their patients. IPAs are often open-panel HMOs.

Operations

The function within pharmaceutical companies charged with handling manufacturing, distribution to wholesalers and other end customers, and procurement of materials and facilities for these activities.

OPPS (Outpatient Prospective Payment System)

The prospective payment system for hospital outpatient departments, established in 2000 to control the cost of services. Under OPPS, hospital outpatient departments receive a predetermined fee per Medicare patient based on the assigned code, an Ambulatory Payment Classification (APC) that groups similar services together.

oral product

A pharmaceutical product meant to be introduced through the mouth in the form of a tablet, capsule, or suspension.

Orange Book

Popular name for the FDA's Compendium of Approved Drug Products with Therapeutic Equivalence Evaluations.

The Orange Book lists all approved drugs, both brand name and generic, prescription and OTC. Physicians and pharmacists can consult the Orange Book to decide whether a generic is an appropriate substitute for a branded drug. This reference also provides information on patents and market exclusivity.

organism

A single, autonomous living thing.

orphan drugs

Drugs for rare diseases and conditions affecting fewer than 200,000 people or a drug that is to be administered to fewer than 200,000 US patients in any given year in the US. To encourage development of treatments for these small markets, Congress passed the Orphan Drug Act of 1983, which grants tax credits and seven years of marketing exclusivity to the pharmaceutical companies that create them.

OTC
See over-the-counter medication.

outcomes research
Evaluates the impact of health care and pharmaceutical interventions on the health consequences (outcomes) in patients and populations. It may also include evaluation of economic variables linked to health outcomes, such as cost-effectiveness or cost-benefit. See pharmacoeconomics and quality of life measures.

out-licensing
Selling rights to use assets or intellectual property by a pharmaceutical or biotech company to a drug it developed and/or owns. The sale may involve a transfer of total ownership or of some more limited interest (e.g., rights to promote and sell a product in certain markets). See co-promotion, co-marketing, and in-licensing.

out-of-pocket costs
The share of health service costs that are borne by the consumer. They include deductibles, co-insurance, co-payments, and full payment for any service not covered by the insurer.

outpatient
Someone receiving medical or surgical care that does not require an overnight stay in the treatment facility. It may be provided in a variety of venues, including a physician office, a clinic, or a hospital.

outsourcing
The trend among pharmaceutical companies toward contracting with outside vendors to provide (some or all of) the functions that a full-service pharmaceutical company would have in-house. Pharmaceutical companies might outsource to CROs (contract research organizations), CMOs (contract manufacturing organizations), CSOs (contract sales organizations), or to full-service CPOs (contract pharmaceutical organizations).

over-the-counter (OTC) medications

Drugs for which prescriptions are not required by federal or state law. Some drugs are marketed from the beginning as OTC products. Other drugs begin as prescription products and eventually shift to OTC status, typically as their patents near expiration.

P

P1, P2, and P3 (Positions 1, 2, and 3)

The predetermined order in which sales representatives are expected to detail products in physician offices. A P1 product, assigned the highest priority, is covered first and in the greatest depth.

package insert (PI)

The document furnished by the manufacturer of a drug and approved by the FDA that describes the drug's chemical structure, its clinical pharmacology, indications and usage, contraindications, warnings and precautions, adverse reactions, overdosage, dosage and administration, and how it is supplied. The PI, in either its complete form (when shipped to pharmacies) or in brief summary form (often when provided to the patient) is folded inside the box containing a drug. Also referred to as the product label, prescribing information, and product information.

packaging

All operations, including filling and labeling, required to transform the manufactured product into a market-ready finished product.

PAI (pre-approval inspection)

An inspection by the FDA of a manufacturing site to verify data submitted in support of an NDA or ANDA and assess compliance with current good manufacturing practices (cGMP). The program covers domestic and foreign manufacturers of both finished dosage form products and APIs.

Also, pure active ingredient.

pallet

A platform with or without sides, on which a number of packages can be loaded for handling by a truck with a fork lift.

palliative treatment

Care that does not alter the course of a disease but alleviates symptoms, such as pain.

pandemic

A worldwide epidemic.

PAR (post-approval research)

Phase 4 studies conducted on a drug after it has won FDA marketing approval for the indication being studied. See post-marketing studies and market expansion studies.

Parallel Track

A policy established in 1990 by the US Public Health Service to speed promising new treatments to AIDS patients. Under this rule, AIDS patients whose conditions do not permit participation in controlled clinical studies can receive investigational drugs that appear promising after initial studies.

parameters

The definition of key attributes of clinical trials, including the population to be included (such attributes as age, gender, and health status), the endpoints to be assessed, the dose(s) to test, and the duration of treatment.

parenteral drug

A drug designed to bypass the gastrointestinal tract. IVs and injections are common parenteral routes of administration. Unlike drugs administered orally or through enteral tubes, which only gradually reach the blood stream, parenteral drugs go directly into a blood vessel, organ, tissue, or lesion.

PAT (process analytical technologies)

An FDA initiative to introduce new manufacturing technologies to the pharmaceutical industry in order to increase efficiency.

patent

In the US, a property right conferred by the US Patent and Trademark Office (USPTO) for a novel and useful invention (in the pharmaceutical context, it might be the active ingredient in a drug or the method of manufacture). The patent holder has sole rights to make, use, and sell the invention during the patent lifetime. In effect, a patent grants the patent holder a limited-period monopoly on the use of the patented property.

patent extension

The right of entities with patented pharmaceutical products to "recover" a portion of the patent life that was consumed by clinical trials and by FDA review of the NDA. This right was created by the Hatch–Waxman Act. A maximum of 5 years can be restored to a patent, and the total remaining patent life cannot exceed 14 years from the product's NDA approval date.

patent filing

An application to the USPTO or a similar international authority for a patent.

patent life

In the pharmaceutical context, the period during which a novel drug or other invention is protected from competitors. In the US, that period is typically 20 years from filing of the patent application; for patents filed or pending in June 1995, the patent life is the greater of 20 years from filing or 17 years from patent grant.

patent prosecution

The USPTO's review of an application to determine whether to grant the patent.

pathogen

Literally, "disease producer." Most frequently used in reference to infectious agents, such as bacteria, viruses, and fungi.

pathological

Related to an abnormality or disease.

pathology

The practice of medicine dealing with the causes and nature of disease and/or death.

patient

A person who requires medical care.

patient advocacy groups

Interest groups for certain diseases (e.g., National Breast Cancer Coalition) or consumer segments (e.g., AARP for older Americans) that lobby for healthcare reform, additional research funding, and or more generous insurance coverage. These advocacy groups are an increasingly powerful force in healthcare.

patient educators

Healthcare professionals (e.g., nurses, counselors, other non-physicians) who provide care instructions to patients and make themselves available to answer any follow-up questions.

patient recruitment

Efforts to enroll subjects in clinical trials. Delays caused by recruitment difficulties are a major clinical development bottleneck.

payers

Corporate entities that provide healthcare coverage, reimbursing or paying claims for healthcare services provided to people they insure. The term includes MCOs, self-insured employers, and government programs such as Medicare and Medicaid.

PBMs (pharmacy benefit management companies)

Organizations that administer drug benefits for payers, including self-insured employers. Typically, these payers "carve out" the outpatient drug benefit (separating it from the medical component of healthcare coverage) and assign responsibility for it to the PBM. Although their role was once limited to claims processing, today they provide such services as contracting with retail pharmacy networks to provide dispensing services at a discount and patient education and/or disease management services to keep drug costs under control.

PCPs (primary care physicians or practitioners)

Physicians whom patients see for routine checkups and general healthcare needs, in contrast to specialists. A term that may encompass pediatricians, family and general practitioners, OB/GYNs, and internists.

PCR (polymerase chain reaction)

A technology developed in the late 1980s that facilitated many significant advances in the diagnosis and monitoring of diseases, such as AIDS and hepatitis. PCR allows minute amounts of genetic material to be amplified (replicated) into billions of copies in just a few hours, facilitating detection of the DNA of pathogenic organisms even before antibodies to these organisms are formed.

PD

See pharmacodynamics.

PDAs (personal digital assistants)

In the pharmaceutical context, handheld electronic tools that offer physicians such functions as online prescribing, drug interaction warnings, lab ordering and result reporting, patient education, and clinical note taking.

PDL (preferred drug list)

See formulary.

PDR (Physicians' Desk Reference(r))

A regularly updated book that provides prescription drug information from the package insert of FDA-approved products. It contains information on indications and usage, administration, dosage, contraindications, dosage, form, clinical pharmacology, precautions, and warnings. Indexed by brand name, manufacturer, product category, and generic and chemical name.

A separate PDR volume is available for nonprescription drugs.

PDUFA

See Prescription Drug User Fee Act.

peak sales

The point in a product's life cycle in which it has reached its maximum anticipated sales volume. The focus of the pharmaceutical company sponsor is to reach peak sales as soon as possible after launch and then to maintain that sales level as long as possible in the face of competition.

peer-reviewed journal

A scholarly publication for which articles are reviewed by outside experts ("peers") in the relevant subject area, who critique the quality of the submission and typically determine whether the material is ultimately published.

peptides

Molecules composed of two or more amino acids, sometimes referred to as the building blocks of proteins. In fact, the difference between proteins and peptides is primarily one of size: Larger peptides are generally referred to as polypeptides or proteins.

persistence

Whether a patient continues to take a drug throughout a period of observation. Along with compliance, persistence is an element of adherence.

Pharmaceutical Research and Manufacturers of America (PhRMA)

The main trade and lobbying group for drug makers in the US, whose stated mission is "to conduct effective advocacy for public policies that encourage discovery of important new medicines for patients by pharmaceutical/biotechnology research companies." Its members include the country's leading research-based pharmaceutical and biotechnology companies. PhRMA works to establish industry codes of conduct in such areas as interactions with potential prescribers.

pharma

Abbreviation for pharmaceutical. Typically used in reference to the industry, rather than the drugs themselves.

pharmaceutical

A drug used as a medicine.

pharmaceutical equivalents

Drugs that they contain the same active ingredient(s), are in the same dosage form, use the same route of administration, and are identical in strength. Two products can be pharmaceutical equivalents even if they differ in attributes such as shape; release mechanism; packaging; excipients; and even, to some extent, labeling.

pharmacists

Licensed professionals who dispense drugs prescribed by physicians and other healthcare practitioners and provide information to patients about medications and their use. They may advise physicians and other health practitioners on the selection, dosage, interactions, and side effects of medications. See PharmD.

pharmacodynamics (PD)

The study of what a drug does to the body. This terminology encompasses, among other things, mechanism of both therapeutic action-the way in which the drug has a beneficial health impact-and mechanism of toxic action for dangerous substances. It also includes the dose-response curve of a drug.

pharmacoeconomics

Study of the costs and consequences (outcomes) associated with the use of pharmaceutical services and drugs. Pharmacoecomics can take into account the overall impact of a pharmaceutical intervention on both overall healthcare costs and quality of life. See outcomes research and quality of life measures.

pharmacogenomics

Efforts to predict the safety, toxicity, or efficacy of drugs in an individual patient or group of patients based on genetic characteristics. Genetic differences are known to affect responses to drug therapy; pharmacogenomics may be able to pinpoint genetically distinct subpopulations for which the efficacy of a drug should be evaluated separately. Additionally, refined understanding of the interaction of particular genes and diseases may lead to new lines of research and new drug therapies.

pharmacokinetics (PK)

What the body does to a drug. Specifically, pharmacokinetics scrutinizes how quickly (and completely) a drug's active ingredient is broken down by the body and delivered to target sites, the byproducts (or metabolites) produced by the breakdown, and the process of elimination from the body. This information, studied through ADME testing, is used to assess drug efficacy and toxicity, as well as appropriate dosing.

pharmacological screening

A phase of discovery in which compounds with diverse chemical structures are tested against a disease-related target in order to anticipate "real world" impact on the human body.

pharmacology

The study of the effects, both beneficial and toxic, of drugs and chemicals on living cells, tissues, organisms. Clinical pharmacology is the study of drugs in man and it is an integral part of pharmacology.

pharmacopeia

A book that lists all drugs and the various factors involved in dispensing them.

Also, the drugs available in a specific pharmacy or specified area.

pharmacotherapeutics

The study of the use of drugs to treat disease. A subcategory of pharmacology.

pharmacovigilance

Monitoring to detect, assess, understand, and prevent adverse effects and other problems related to drug therapy.

pharmacy

A place where drugs are dispensed. Types of pharmacies include retail chains, independents, Internet and mail-order, and hospital and clinic.

pharmacy aides

Clerks or cashiers whose primary duties include answering the phone, ringing up sales, and stocking shelves. They often work closely with pharmacy technicians.

pharmacy benefit

Coverage of specified prescription drugs by an insurance company. Often, beneficiaries will have an identification card documenting their eligibility and will have to cover some of the drug cost themselves through co-payments, deductibles, or co-insurance. Also referred to as a prescription drug benefit, although it sometimes includes non-prescription drugs.

pharmacy costs

Term that MCOs and PBMs use for the costs they incur when enrollees obtain drugs on an outpatient basis. "Pharmaceutical costs" is not employed because expenses incurred include charges for pharmacy dispensing.

pharmacy directors

The healthcare professionals employed by payers, PBMs, and providers such as hospitals to guide decisions regarding appropriate formulary status and drug coverage. Pharmacy directors are prominent members of the P&T committees at these organizations.

In a retail pharmacy setting, the pharmacy director is manager of the team of pharmacists and pharmacy technicians employed at that site or perhaps by an entire chain.

pharmacy technician

A non-pharmacist who works under the supervision of a pharmacist, assisting with routine activities, such as counting tablets and labeling bottles for prescriptions, entering prescription information into a computer, and assisting with inventory control. Technicians refer all questions regarding prescriptions, drug information, and health matters to a pharmacist. Their duties are typically more complex than those of a pharmacy aide.

PharmD

Doctor of Pharmacy degree–the advanced degree for pharmacists. A PharmD requires four years of professional study, following a minimum of two years of pre-pharmacy study, for a total of six academic years following high school.

phase 1 (or I) trials

Initial clinical studies to determine the metabolism and pharmacological actions of drugs in humans, side effects associated with increasing doses, and to gain early evidence of efficacy. Studies are conducted in a small number of healthy volunteers and/or patients.

phase 2 (or II) trials

Typically the first clinical trials in which a drug is given to people with the disease it is intended to treat–and the first studies using a control group. Varied dosing levels are assessed for tolerance, short-term side effects, and efficacy. The goal by the end of phase 2 is to generate proof of concept (that the drug is efficacious for its intended use).

These trials, which usually involve on no more than a few hundred patients, are also used to refine the protocol for the large-scale phase 3 studies, including characteristics of the patients to be included, appropriate endpoints for assessing efficacy, and appropriate dose.

phase 3 (or III) trials

Essentially a larger-scale version of phase 2 trials, in which several hundred to thousands of patients (often in countries across the globe) with the relevant disease participate. Phase 3 clinical trials measure the impact of the drug on key endpoints defined during phase 2 and monitor the drug for adverse effects.

Data from these trials are used to settle the question of whether the drug's benefits outweigh its risks and to define appropriate product labeling, populations in which the drug should not be used, and adverse interactions with foods and other drugs. At some point during phase 3, the NDA for any promising product is submitted to the FDA.

Such clinical trials are usually randomized, double-blind, controlled studies to eliminate bias to the extent possible.

phase 3a (or IIIa) trials

Phase 3 trials that occur before NDA submission.

phase 3b (or IIIb) trials

Phase 3 trials that occur after NDA submission but before FDA approval and launch.

phase 4 (or IV) trials

Post-marketing studies (i.e., after NDA approval), conducted to either gather additional safety and efficacy data for marketing purposes or to satisfy conditions specified by the FDA in granting approval.

Issues that may be examined include the efficacy and other attributes of the drug compared with its competitors, the drug's long-term effectiveness and the incidence of adverse reactions/events (also referred to as post-marketing surveillance), the efficacy of new formulations and dosing regimens, and/or other possible uses (indications) for the drug-new populations that might benefit from it. Such trials are sometimes called post-approval research (PAR) or post-marketing studies. When their goal is to assess additional populations for whom the drug might prove beneficial, they may be called market expansion studies.

phenotype

A set of observable physical characteristics of an individual organism, including a person. The traits may be physical, biochemical, or physiologic (that is, related to the function of the body or a constituent tissue or organ). Phenotype may be the outcome of a combination of genotype, environment, and lifestyle.

A common but less strictly correct use of phenotype is as a synonym for a single trait, such as blonde hair.

PHO (physician-hospital organization)

A joint venture between physicians and a hospital, primarily for the purpose of negotiating favorable contracts with insurers and employers by offering the advantage of a unified network of inpatient and outpatient services.

PhRMA

See Pharmaceutical Research and Manufacturers of America.

physician assistant (PA)

A mid-level healthcare professional who works under the supervision of a licensed doctor (an MD) or osteopathic physician (a DO). His/her responsibilities vary based on training and state law. Typically, the PA sees many of the same types of patients as the supervising physician does, but the more complicated or non-routine cases are referred to the physician. PAs can prescribe medications independently in most states in the US. All states require that new PAs complete an accredited, formal education program. A PA must have at least a bachelor's degree and many have a master's degree.

physician contingency reserve

The percentage of an MCO payment for physician services that is withheld until the end of the year as an incentive for appropriate utilization and quality of care. The reserve is ultimately paid out by the MCO, or retained, based upon review of physician cost effectiveness.

physician dispensing

Physician provision of a drug directly to a patient-without the involvement of a pharmacy. Examples include vaccines and the initial dose of a medication that a sales representative has supplied as a sample.

physician profiling

Regular reports on the cost and resource utilization practices of individual physicians, which are usually compared with norms in the same specialty. These reports are typically used by MCOs and hospitals to encourage physicians to bring their cost and utilization into line with those of their peers. Pharmaceutical companies also use physician profiling to aid in targeting high prescribers as part of their sales efforts.

physician promotion

Pharmaceutical promotions targeted at physicians such as samples, journal ads, and speaker programs.

physicians

Healthcare professionals with an MD (Doctor of Medicine) or DO (Doctor of Osteopathy) licensed within by a state to practice medicine and prescribe drugs.

PI

Principal investigator or package insert, depending on the context.

pilot manufacturing facilities

Manufacturing plants where low-volume quantities of a drug formulation are produced for use during early clinical development.

pipeline forecasts

Forecasts of the number and sales value of products that will emerge from R&D over a certain time frame.

pivotal trials

Phase 3 clinical trials (usually randomized, controlled, and double-blind) that provide evidence of a drug's efficacy and are therefore deemed successful (pivotal). Normally, two pivotal trials are required to ensure the validity of the studies, although if the results are extremely strong, one may suffice.

placebo

An inactive (dummy) substance that looks exactly the same as, and is administered in the same way as, the study drug in a clinical trial. Placebo is sometimes referred to as a "sugar pill." It is used for comparative purposes in assessing adverse events and efficacy of an investigational drug. No sick participant receives a placebo in a clinical trial, however, if there is a known effective treatment available. In that case, the standard treatment would be used as the comparator in the clinical trial.

placebo-controlled study

A clinical trial in which one group of participants receives an inactive substance ("sugar pill"), while the other group receives the drug being tested. The results from the two groups are then compared to ascertain whether the investigational drug is more effective in treating the disease or condition.

plan

See health plan.

platelets

Disk-shaped blood cells that stick to the edges of wounds, promoting blood clotting and temporarily covering the wound.

platform technology

Any technique or tool that facilitates efforts to work out complex, high-value solutions; for instance, the operating system of your computer is a platform technology and, in pharmaceutical research, any innovative methodology that generates new compounds, such as combinatorial chemistry, is a platform technology. Genomics and proteomics are sometimes described as a state-of-the-art platform technologies for identifying disease markers and for drug discovery and development.

PMPM (per member per month)

The most common structure of payments that employers and other corporate entities make to MCOs and other insurers in exchange for healthcare coverage. This system of payment is known as "capitation," because payments are calculated on a per capita basis, not based upon actual service utilization in any month. (PMPM rates take into account historical usage patterns and may be adjusted based upon actuarial factors such as age and sex.)

PMPY (per member per year)

An alternative to PMPM for structuring payments for insurance coverage.

POA (plan of action)

A detailed roadmap for translating Marketing strategy into Sales operations.

point-of-sale (POS)

The pharmacy in which a consumer picks up a prescription.

point-of-sale edit

Edits set up by a health plan that are processed when the claim is submitted electronically by a pharmacy. Some edits provide pharmacists with dispensing instructions. They may also recommend that the pharmacist advocate use of a generic or alternative brand.

POSs (point-of-service plans)

Least restrictive form of MCO plan, sometimes referred to an open-ended or open-model HMO. For each episode of care, patients are free to choose any service provider, in or out of network. The care will be reimbursed regardless of provider, although the co-payment and/or deductible is higher for providers outside the plan network. (Some POSs also have tiered in-network rates based on whether the provider is within the narrower HMO network or a broader PPO network.)

post-marketing studies

Phase 4 studies of drugs that have already obtained marketing approval from the FDA. They may be mandated by the FDA to obtain more information about the safety of a drug; to assess the incidence of a specific adverse drug reaction; or, if the drug was approved based on surrogate endpoints, to prove the drug produces an actual clinical benefit.

Pharmaceutical companies may also choose to pursue such studies even if none are mandated by the FDA, in order to develop more robust data for product positioning purposes or to identify additional potential indications. See market expansion studies, phase 4 trials, and seeding studies.

post-market surveillance or post-marketing surveillance

The FDA's system of ongoing scrutiny of marketed drugs to identify any serious safety issues that weren't apparent during clinical trials. Under its adverse drug reporting system, pharmaceutical companies must report all serious and unexpected adverse experiences associated with their drugs within 15 days. Feedback to the FDA from physicians and other healthcare professionals, as well as consumers, is purely voluntary, although the FDA has established the MedWatch system to encourage such reporting.

potentiation

The increase in the therapeutic or toxic effect of one drug through the administration of another drug.

PPM or PPMC (physician practice management corporation)

An organization that provides financial, administrative, and purchasing services to physician practices in order to increase the cost-efficiency of operations. Some PPMs actually purchase the physician practices to which they provide this infrastructure support.

PPO (preferred provider organization)

A form of MCO in which members have access to a large network of providers. PPOs offer members greater choice than HMOs. Network providers agree to accept discounted payments and adhere to certain utilization procedures.

PPS (Prospective Payment System)

The system under which Medicare or Medicaid pays hospitals for most in-patient care, which is based on predefined DRG rates. Because payment per care episode is usually the same regardless of resource consumption (that is, payment reflects a forecast of what the cost should be, based on aggregate hospital historical data and care guidelines), hospitals have an incentive to enhance their profits-or, at least, avoid losses-by making operations efficient and controlling utilization of expensive drugs and other resources.

P&T committees (Pharmacy and Therapeutics committees)

A group of physicians, pharmacists, and other relevant experts that advise an MCO, PBM, hospital or other institution regarding safe and cost-effective medications to include on a formulary.

practice guidelines

Also known as practice parameters or medical protocols, they are care instructions that have been tested through studies of clinical outcomes and found to produce the best results. Each guideline tells the caregiver which treatment options (or even which specific steps) are advisable, given a particular set of symptoms and/or lab test results.

pre-authorization or prior authorization

The requirement that a physician obtain advance permission from the patient's health plan to use or prescribe a drug. If such permission is not obtained—either because it wasn't sought or because utilization review personnel didn't consider the drug clinically necessary—the plan will not reimburse use of the drug. Prior-authorization requirements are most frequently used for drugs that are disfavored because of their expense compared with similarly effective alternatives.

pre-certification

The requirement that a provider/enrollee obtain advance permission from the covering health plan for a hospital admission (either inpatient or outpatient). The provider or the enrollee will suffer payment penalties if precertification is not obtained.

Also known as "precert."

pre-clinical development

The testing of a compound in the lab and in animals that precedes testing in humans (clinical trials).

The overall purpose of pre-clinical testing is to determine whether the product is safe enough to test on humans and shows sufficient therapeutic promise to justify commercial development.

Efficacy and toxicity are assessed. Through ADME testing in animals, bioavailability is determined and the best delivery method is identified. The manufacturing methodology for the drug is also defined at this stage.

pre-clinical research

See pre-clinical development.

pre-clinical testing

See pre-clinical development.

predictive modeling

A statistical process by which a clinical database is used to describe mathematically the likelihood of outcomes, given a set of data values of predictor variables. For instance, blood cholesterol levels, family history, and characteristics such as height and weight can be used to predict the risk of heart disease or stroke. The process can also be used to estimate the probable impact of treatment and lifestyle modification on that risk.

preferred drug

Favorable formulary status that health plans usually accord to drugs for which they have negotiated a rebate contract. The favorable status usually translates into a lower co-payment than for alternative products.

prescribers

Physicians and, depending upon state regulations, nurse practitioners, pharmacists, and physician assistants who have the legal authority to write a prescription for a drug.

prescribing information

See package insert.

prescription drug or prescription medication

A drug that has been approved by the FDA, which either federal or state law restricts by requiring a licensed healthcare professional (typically a physician) to fill out a prescription.

Prescription Drug Marketing Act of 1987 (PDMA)

A US law enacted to reduce the risk that prescription drugs that are counterfeit, adulterated, or expired will be sold to the American public. It banned the sale, purchase, or trade of drug samples and drug coupons; banned reimportation of prescription drugs produced in the US, except when reimported to the manufacturer or for emergency use; and required state licensure of wholesale distributors of prescription drugs. As a result of PDMA, physicians cannot sell the free samples they receive from pharmaceutical companies, and pharmaceutical companies must rigorously track samples distributed and collect unused ones.

Prescription Drug User Fee Act of 1992 (PDUFA)

A US law under which drug manufacturers were required to pay user fees to fund the hire of additional FDA reviewers in order to speed the NDA review process.

prevalence

The total number of cases (both new and existing) of a defined condition (e.g., a disease or other health-related event) in a specific population during a specified period of time, usually expressed as a percentage. Hypothetical example: "The prevalence of asthma in the US is 6%." Chronic or life-long diseases, such as diabetes, tend to have a higher prevalence than acute illnesses, such as flu, which can have a high annual incidence but low prevalence. By contrast, see incidence.

primary care

In health systems that use primary care physicians (PCPs) as gatekeepers who must provide referrals to other health services, interactions with those PCPs.

In systems that allow direct access to specialists without referral, the distinction is usually based on treatment facility-clinics and physician offices are considered primary care and standard hospital services are considered secondary care.

primary care physicians

See PCPs.

primary endpoint

The main result or primary outcome that is measured at the end of a study to see if a given treatment was effective (e.g., in a cancer treatment study, the difference in survival between the treatment group and the control group). The primary endpoint is decided before the study begins and is clearly identified in the study protocol. A study may also have a secondary endpoint, which allows investigation of subsidiary questions that, while scientifically important, do not have the same priority of clinical interest in the patient group being studied.

primary packaging

The packaging that physically touches a product and is expected to provide the greatest protection of its purity, potency, and integrity. For drugs, that would include the multi-dose foil pack known as a blister pack or the bottle in which tablets or pills are typically enclosed.

primary care products

Products that are typically prescribed on an outpatient basis by a patient's primary care physician-a general or family practitioner, internist, OB/GYN, or pediatrician. Pharmaceutical companies distinguish these products from specialty products, which are typically prescribed by physicians with narrower fields of expertise, such as oncology or cardiology. Many companies have separate sales forces for primary care and specialty products.

primary research

Unmediated sources of information that provide the reader/observer with an opportunity to analyze raw data. The category includes questionnaires and surveys and the publication of original study findings by study leaders. It does not include a survey article summarizing multiple past studies.

Primary research is sometimes called original research.

principal investigator

The healthcare professional, typically a physician, responsible for the overall conduct of the clinical trial at a particular site. As part of the site selection process, the PI's academic credentials and expertise are scrutinized. Principal investigator is a regulatory term of art that carries with it specific responsibilities for study conduct.

prior authorization

See pre-authorization or prior authorization.

priority drugs

A category created by the FDA to clarify the speed with which NDA review should be completed.

Under the Food and Drug Administration Modernization Act (FDAMA), reviews for NDAs are designated as either standard or priority. The target date for FDA review for a priority drug is 6 months. The target for a standard drug is 10 months.

CBER and CDER have different standards for granting priority review. CBER requires potentially significant improvement in the safety and effectiveness of the treatment for a serious or life-threatening disease. CDER will grant priority review to any product that represents a significant improvement over current treatment, regardless of whether the disease is serious or life-threatening.

private insurer

A non-government entity that provides health insurance benefits, including Blue Cross and Blue Shield plans, commercial insurers, and managed care plans.

private label

A "house brand" OTC drug (e.g., from Walgreens), which usually sells for less than the equivalent national brand.

private practice

The structure of most physician practices in the US. Physicians in private practice are self-employed or employed by a group practice in which they have an ownership stake, rather than employed by an outside organization, such as a staff-model HMO or hospital.

procurement

The process of obtaining supplies and services. In the pharmaceutical context, this typically refers to obtaining raw materials for manufacturing and packaging, but can also include purchases for other business supplies and services. The term can also refer to the federal government's process for obtaining adequate supplies of pharmaceuticals.

product claim ads

Drug ads regulated by the FDA that include both the name of a product and its intended indication, or make a healthcare claim about a prescription drug. Claims of drug benefits, such as safety and effectiveness, must be balanced with disclosure of risks and limitations. This even-handed presentation is referred to as fair balance. When such ads are in print, sponsors must provide a brief summary of risk information included in the product's FDA-approved label. Broadcast product claim ads have to offer convenient access to the approved label (e.g., an 800 number or Web site). The phrase "adequate provision" is used to describe the convenient access option for broadcast ads.

product label

See label.

product monograph

A factual, non-promotional, scientific document on the drug product that describes the properties, claims, indications, and conditions of use for the drug. It also contains other information that may be required for optimal, safe, and effective use of the drug. Product monographs are used internally in a pharmaceutical company for training and reference purposes, and also may be distributed to potential prescribers by sales reps and MSLs, particularly around product launch. Product monographs, however, must meet FDA (specifically DDMAC) standards regarding promotional materials if they are to be distributed externally to customers.

positioning

Translation of a product's overall value proposition into highly specific messages regarding attributes of particular interest to target customer segments, including prescribers, consumers, and payers.

promotion plan

The plan developed by Marketing for a specific product, which includes approved messages that will be used in promotion (the message plan) and defines the means of delivering those messages to target customers (channels and techniques, known as the promotional mix).

promotional mix

The channels (e.g., sales force visits, print ads, Internet sites) and the techniques used to disseminate product value messages to key customers.

promotional spending

Expenditure on advertising and other means of reaching prescribers, payers, and consumers. Sometimes referred to as promotional spend.

promotions

Any materials issued by or on behalf of a company-or any events sponsored by or on behalf of a company-that mention one or more products.

proof of concept

Preliminary evidence, based on phase 2 clinical trials, that a compound is effective for its intended purpose.

prophylactic

A drug, vaccine, lifestyle management approach, or other intervention designed to prevent the onset of a disease or condition.

prospective study

A study that is carefully designed in advance to be carried out on a specific population in a controlled environment. In other words, a study in which people are initially enrolled and their medical progress is tracked going forward. By contrast, see retrospective study.

protein

A large, complex molecule composed of amino acids. Proteins play a critical role in the functioning-and malfunctioning-of the body. In a process known as gene expression, our genetic makeup (including any mutations) is translated into action through protein synthesis. Many pharmaceuticals attempt either to inhibit harmful protein activity or stimulate essential protein activity. Key proteins include enzymes, hormones, and antibodies.

proteome

All the proteins produced by a genome (that is, an organism's DNA) and their interactions. Because genetic makeup dictates the proteins produced, the proteome can be thought of as a manifestation of the genome.

proteomics

An effort to catalogue the proteins expressed by a cell or tissue-and how they interact. This information can be used to study the way diseases operate at the protein level.

protocol

See clinical protocol.

protocol-driven treatment

Care delivery defined by highly specific, generally highly complex step-by-step guidelines. Oncology and AIDS treatments are both protocol-driven.

provider network

See network.

providers

The personnel and institutions licensed to offer healthcare services, including physicians, nurses, pharmacists, pharmacies, hospitals, and skilled nursing facilities.

psychometrics

Quantitative measures of psychological well-being or particular aspects of human behavior, such as personality, motivation, values, interests or other attributes.

PTO (US Patent and Trade Office)

The regulatory agency that grants US patents for products/concepts that are both unique and useful. Among other things, the PTO grants US patents to pharmaceutical companies. See USPTO.

Public Health Service (PHS)

One of the Federal Markets customer segments. The agency responsible for the health of the American people, which oversees agencies including the FDA, CDC, and NIH.

pull-through

Prescriptions and sales of a promoted pharmaceutical product, as opposed to reimbursement and access, which simply means that drugs will be covered by payers (in whole or part) if utilized. Field Sales takes primary responsibility for driving pull-through.

Q

qualitative research or studies

Information collected regarding the motivations, attitudes, and behaviors of respondents in a given situation.

QA (quality assurance)

A function within pharmaceutical companies and biotechs that monitors compliance with GMPs and the process specifications approved by the FDA in the NDA filing. In short, QA ensures process integrity and compliance with GMP. QA verifies that each batch is created following the recipe or formula and the production process approved by the FDA.

QC (quality control)

The function within pharmaceutical companies and biotechs that checks to make sure that compliance with process standards such as GCP and GMP actually produces the high-quality results intended. QC, in short, ensures the integrity of outcomes. In the manufacturing context, QC samples and conducts lab tests of raw materials and products to ensure that the production process actually yields a homogeneous product that meets NDA specifications.

Quality (function)

A group (or two separate groups) within a pharmaceutical company or biotech with QA and QC responsibilities.

quality-adjusted life year

A unit of measure for health outcomes, in which the number of years a patient survives in impaired health are "discounted" by reference to the same number of years in full health.

quality-of-life measures

Patient outcome measures that extend beyond traditional measures of mortality and morbidity to include such dimensions as physical and social function, limitations due to physical or emotional problems, mental health, energy, pain, and general health perceptions. The most commonly used instrument to measure health-related quality of life is the SF-36, which is sometimes administered in clinical trials to assess the effect of a pharmaceutical treatment on patients' quality of life. See SF-36.

quantitative research or quantitative studies

Type of research or study that examines phenomena through the numerical representation of observations and statistical analysis, as distinct from qualitative research. Questionnaires or surveys are frequently used in this type of research.

R

RAM (regional account manager)

An account manager in a pharmaceutical company that organizes managed markets outreach on a regional rather than a national basis.

randomization

A method of assigning patients in clinical trials to different treatment groups. Once a pool of appropriate candidates for a trial is established, randomization (rather than, for instance, investigator choice) is employed in designating patients as members of either the control or the test group. This approach eliminates selection bias that might undermine the reliability of comparisons between the two groups.

rational drug design

The engineering of drugs based on the structure of the intended protein target. Because proteins have a complex three-dimensional structure, super-computers are employed to facilitate the design process. This approach is an alternative to the time-consuming process of synthesizing large numbers of compounds (or finding them in nature) and screening them for efficacy against a given disease.

RBCs (red blood cells)

Cells containing a protein chemical called hemoglobin, which transport oxygen and carry away carbon dioxide throughout the body.

RCT

Randomized, controlled trial

reagent

A chemical substance known to react in a specific manner that can therefore be used to detect or produce another substance. Reagents are sometimes used to manufacture a drug substance.

rebates

In the pharmaceutical industry, the term (used interchangeably with charge-backs) refers to the discount off standard pricing that pharmaceutical companies grant favored MCOs or PBMs in order to obtain a favorable formulary position.

A discount provided to a customer after purchase from a wholesaler or retailer.

receptor

A protein in a cell or on a cell membrane that can serve as a binding site for antigens, antibodies, or other cellular or immunological components. Most drugs act on receptors-structures that fit, in a "lock and key" fashion, with the drug being administered. The interaction of drug and receptor produces the desired beneficial effect.

The names given receptors often reflect the chemical or compound that trigger intracellular changes influencing the behavior of cells (e.g., a histamine receptor).

recipe

The formula, including process steps and ingredients, used to manufacture a drug.

recombinant DNA (rDNA)

DNA which has been altered by joining genetic material from two different sources. It usually involves insertion of a gene from one organism into the genome of a different organism, generally of a different species.

Red Book

Formally the Drug Topics Red Book. An annual reference work containing pricing information for prescription and over-the-counter products, NDC numbers for FDA-approved drugs, and Orange Book codes reflecting FDA evaluations of therapeutic equivalence.

reference drug pricing

A cost-sharing strategy commonly used to control drug expenditures, in which a benefit plan fully reimburses prescription drugs that are equally or less expensive than the reference price, and requires patients to pay the extra cost of therapeutically equivalent but higher priced drugs.

reference listed drug (RLD)

A drug approved by the FDA as a brand upon which a generic manufacturer relies in submitting an ANDA request-that is, the brand to which the generic claims to be bioequivalent.

referral

A recommendation from a patient's primary care physician (PCP) that a specialist be consulted or certain other expensive health services be utilized. The PCP acts as a gatekeeper on behalf of the patient's health plan, which may not reimburse such services without the referral.

refusal-to-file letter

This response from the FDA to an NDA or BLA filing indicates major deficiencies in the application and gives the applicant the opportunity to amend the application so that a complete review can be conducted by FDA.

refractory

Resistant to initial or standard treatment.

regulation

An authoritative rule having the force of law that implement government program. For instance, the FDA develops specific regulations to carry out its duties as outlined in various pieces of federal legislation.

Regulatory Affairs (function)

A function within a pharmaceutical company that handles interactions with governmental regulatory bodies-primarily the FDA-and ensures that drug development, manufacturing, and marketing efforts comply with governmental rules. Each drug sponsor has a Regulatory Affairs department that manages the drug approval process.

regulatory review period

Time period during which a drug undergoes a testing phase (in humans) and an approval phase. For drugs evaluated by CDER, it runs from the effective date of the Investigational New Drug Application (IND) through to approval (if granted) of the New Drug Application (NDA). If the regulatory review period has been extraordinarily long, the drug manufacturer may be granted a patent extension, through a cooperative effort of the Patent and Trademark Office (PTO) and the FDA.

reimbursement and access

In the pharmaceutical industry, this term refers to whether a drug will be covered by a third-party payer (e.g., insurer, the government, MCO) and whether a patient has the ability to obtain medical care or medications. Pharmaceutical companies, particularly Managed Markets departments, are understandably concerned about reimbursement and access issues, as they affect profitability of their products. See access.

reimportation

The re-introduction to the US market of US-made prescription drugs that had been sent to foreign countries. Many elderly people in the US seek out reimported drugs because the prices in other countries are lower. Pharmaceutical companies generally oppose reimportation. Controversy exists as to whether such reimported drugs can be verified as safe and genuine.

reminder ads

Ads regulated by the FDA that disclose the name of the product and certain specific descriptive information such as dosage form (i.e., tablet, capsule, or syrup), but do not specify the product's indication (use) or make any claims or representations about the product. The regulations specifically exempt "reminder" ads from the risk disclosure requirements. Such ads are not allowed, however, for products with serious warnings (called "black box" warnings) in their label (package insert).

research and development (R&D)

The process of identifying and testing the safety and efficacy of new compounds or new uses (indications) for existing compounds. The research and development process includes drug discovery and clinical development.

research-based pharmaceutical companies

Companies that perform original research resulting in the development and marketing of branded ethical products.

resistance (drug)

The reduction in effectiveness (or total ineffectiveness) of previously successful treatments for an infection due to mutations in the microbes (organisms) that cause that infection.

resident

A physician who has graduated from medical school but is undergoing additional training in his or her specialty. Most specialties require at least three years of residency training, and many specialties require four years or more. Even after completing their residencies, physicians may undertake fellowships for further specialty training.

residency

Up to seven years of graduate medical education in a specific medical specialty following medical school graduation. Training occurs in accredited hospitals, clinics, and other healthcare facilities where resident physicians work under the supervision of physicians who are recognized as experts in their chosen specialty or subspecialty.

respite care

Short-term health services offered to provide a "breather" to members of the immediate family or any other unpaid primary caregiver. Respite care can include such services as home healthcare and adult day care.

retail chain

A group of affiliated retail pharmacies, typically national or regional in geographic scope. Examples include Eckerd, CVS, and Walgreens. Some pharmacy chains are part of mass-merchant chains (e.g., Target).

retail pharmacy

A pharmacy that will dispense drugs to any customer with a prescription—not simply those who are patients of a particular provider or members of a particular health plan. Such pharmacies may be independent or part of a retail chain.

retrospective study

A review of previous clinical experiences of patients with a particular condition or disease, in order to collect information on the efficacy of a particular intervention (for instance, a drug). Such research often involves analysis of patient medical records and claims data. By contrast, see prospective study.

RFID (radio frequency identification technology) tags

Electronic tags that are in experimental use in pharmaceutical supply chain management. They are attached to drug cases and pallets to track them. One purpose is to prevent drug counterfeiting.

RFP (request for proposal)

A document used to solicit vendor bids for the provision of goods or services. For instance, pharmaceutical companies send RFPs to CROs inviting them to submit bids for drug development work.

ride-alongs

Sales calls (particularly physician office visits) in which a junior sales representative is accompanied by a sales manager or more senior sales representative. Their purpose is to train and evaluate the performance of the less experienced sales representative.

risk-benefit ratio

The risk of a drug to users, weighed against its potential benefits, usually used in relation to subjecting patients to unnecessary risk.

risk sharing

Contractual relationships in which the parties share the burden of higher-than-expected costs. While risk-sharing contracts are most common between MCOs and providers, they are also sometimes entered into by pharmaceutical companies and the MCOs that grant favored status to their brands. The pharmaceutical companies agree to bear some of the excess cost if a brand does not prove to be as cost-effective as anticipated (that is, if patients do not recover as quickly as expected or face unforeseen complications).

RN

Registered nurse. RNs are state certified and must have a two-year associate degree, a three-year degree , or a four-year baccalaureate.

RNA (ribonucleic acid)

A chemical found in cells that plays an important role in the synthesis of proteins and in other cellular activities. The structure of RNA is similar to that of DNA, except that it is usually single- and not double-stranded.

RNA molecules come in a number of different forms, each with a different function. They include messenger RNA (mRNA), transfer RNA, and ribosomal RNA.

route of administration

The means by which a drug is administered, including oral methods (liquid, tablets, capsules), injections (subcutaneous, intravenous, intramuscular), inhalation (via aerosol or dry powder inhalers, nasal sprays), transdermal patch, sublingual absorption (placed under tongue), and topical and rectal options. See also delivery mechanism.

RSD (regional sales director)

In the Sales hierarchy, the people who manage district managers (DMs).

RUG (Resource Utilization Group)

Classification system for nursing home patients that the federal government and some states use to define appropriate reimbursement levels.

Rx

Shorthand for prescription. It may be derived from the Latin word for "recipe."

S

Sales (function)

A commercial function within a pharmaceutical company or CSO whose primary customer targets are prescribers (that is, physicians and to a lesser extent nurse practitioners, physician assistants, and pharmacists). The position of the Sales function varies by company. In a typical midsize pharmaceutical company, a vice president of Sales or national sales director typically heads the field force.

sales force automation (SFA)

See SFA.

sales force structure

The strategic organization of a sales force in order to optimize the cost-efficiency of outreach to high-priority customers. Typical structuring principles include geography, therapeutic area, and target customer base (e.g., specialists versus primary care customers).

Sales Operations (function)

Headquarters infrastructure for the pharmaceutical company sales force. Its scope often includes sales force training, IT support (the SFA system), and the development of sales force incentive compensation schemes.

sales representatives

The group within the Sales function that pays calls on physician offices and details products. The pharmaceutical sales representative is the public face of the company. In every practice environment-physician office, hospital, or clinic-the representative's responsibility is to influence prescribing behavior. A sales representative may present only primary care products or only specialty products-or present the company's entire product portfolio to institutional customers or MCOs.

samples

In the context of sales force calls to physician offices, hospitals, and pharmacies, the "starter kits" of a product that are provided free of charge to encourage use. Free samples are one of the largest promotional expenses incurred by pharmaceutical companies. Pharmaceutical company sales representatives are responsible for keeping careful track of the samples they distribute.

scale-up (or scaling up)

Increasing the batch size of drugs for purposes of clinical trials and ultimately commercial marketing. During pre-clinical development, the manufacturing methodology for a drug is defined in the laboratory and tested in pilot manufacturing facilities. As a compound passes successfully through various phases of clinical trials, production is scaled up until it reaches a volume appropriate for commercial sale.

scheduled drug

A drug whose use and distribution is tightly controlled because of its potential for abuse. Scheduled drugs are classified under the Controlled Substances Act (CSA), part of the Comprehensive Drug Abuse Prevention and Control Act of 1970. The CSA places all substances regulated under federal law into one of five schedules based upon medicinal value, harmfulness, and potential for abuse or addiction. Schedule I is reserved for the most dangerous drugs that have no recognized medical use, while Schedule V is used for those drugs with the lowest abuse potential.

The CSA creates a closed system of distribution for those authorized to handle controlled substances. The cornerstone of this system is the registration of all those authorized by the DEA to handle controlled substances. All individuals and firms that are registered by the DEA to handle controlled substance must maintain accurate inventories and transfer records.

For a synonymous term, see controlled substances.

scientific rationale

In the context of the pharmaceutical industry, a credible and scientific explanation of how and/or why a drug or treatment regimen works, usually to improve human health. The FDA requires a discussion of the clinical rationale for a drug as part of a pharmaceutical company's NDA filing. See also clinical rationale.

script

Shorthand term for prescription. Also, scrip.

secondary care

Outpatient services from specialists and hospital care, both inpatient and outpatient. In non-emergency situations, access often requires a referral from a PCP.

secondary packaging

The outer package into which primary packaging is placed, such as a folding carton. The main purpose of secondary packaging is to protect the product during shipping and distribution, provide essential information, and present an attractive, distinctive brand image.

secondary research

Analyses/syntheses of the original work (e.g., interviews, surveys, clinical trials) of others. This category includes "survey" articles summarizing findings from multiple studies.

second-line therapy

Drugs utilized only when the preferred initial form of treatment (the first-line therapy) has failed, or in patients for whom the first-line therapy is for some reason inappropriate (e.g., carries unusually high risks).

second-stage drug

A synonym for second-line therapy.

Section 340B

A part of the Public Health Service Act enacted in 1992, which requires pharmaceutical manufacturers participating in the Medicaid program to provide discounts on covered outpatient drugs purchased by specified government-supported facilities, called "covered entities," which serve vulnerable populations. The amount of these discounts is comparable to the best price discounts to which Medicaid is entitled under the 1990 rebate program; however, covered entities are free to negotiate even deeper discounts than the best price.

The definition of "covered entities" includes thousands of facilities specified by the Public Health Service, including selected hospitals, family planning clinics, public housing primary care clinics, and homeless clinics.

seeding studies

Phase 4 studies evaluating newly approved drugs, usually through office-based medical practices. The primary purpose of these studies is to expose a greater number of prescribers and patients to the new product. Physicians are frequently given free samples of the newly approved drug and asked to track its effect in their patients. Such studies have been controversial, as some claim they are purely a promotional tactic and not clinical research.

service area

The geographic area from which a health plan accepts members. For plans that require members to use only in-network providers, it is also the area where services are provided. Plan members who leave the service area may be disenrolled.

segmentation

The division of a population (e.g., patients, physicians) into distinct groups based upon some agreed-upon criterion or criteria. Deciling is a segmentation method commonly used in the pharmaceutical industry.

selection bias

Potential error introduced into a study by the selection of different types of people into treatment and comparison groups. As a result, differences in outcomes between groups could potentially result from pre-existing differences between the groups, rather than from the treatment itself. Randomization is employed to eliminate the possibility of selection bias.

selectivity

The ability of a therapeutic dose of a drug to affect its intended target without affecting other parts of the body. Selectivity is generally desirable in a drug, e.g., it is desirable that an antibacterial agent kill bacteria without harming host cells. By contrast, see specificity.

In the realm of diagnostic testing, sensitivity represents the ability to avoid "false negatives"-the failure to identify persons with a disease as having that disease.

self-report instrument

A survey or questionnaire that patients are asked to fill out to record their perspective on measures of well-being, such as mood, pain level, and ability to pursue/enjoy normal life activities. Such instruments are used to assess the impact of a drug or other intervention in areas that are difficult to assess objectively. The SF–36 is one type of self-report instrument, but myriad variants exist.

self-warehousing

Transportation and storage of surplus drug supplies in owned facilities by entities (e.g., retail chains) that have traditionally relied upon wholesalers for storage.

sequelae

Abnormal conditions or diseases that follow and are usually caused by a previous illness.

sequencing

Determination of the order of nucleotides of a DNA or RNA molecule.

serious adverse event (SAE)

Any adverse event (AE) that is fatal, life-threatening, or permanently disabling, or requires hospitalization.

severity of illness

Levels of disease progression or seriousness among patients with the same diagnosis.

SFA (sales force automation)

The use of specialized software to automate sales activities, including contact management, information sharing, customer management, and sales forecast analysis. SFA is often used interchangeably with CRM, but CRM does not necessarily involve automation of sales activities.

In the pharmaceutical context, SFA allows sales reps to enter and receive complete, timely information about characteristics of target physicians (including their preferences and the decile into which they fall for prescriptions of various types of products) and recent and planned sales activity directed to those physicians.

SF-36 (Short Form 36)

A type of self-report instrument in which patients record subjective assessments of their quality of life. Developed for the Medical Outcomes Study, this health status questionnaire can be used to assess the functioning and well-being of patients with any chronic disease. Eight dimensions are covered: physical function; social function; role limitations due to physical problems; role limitations due to emotional problems; mental health; energy/vitality; pain; and general health perception.

The SF-36 is scored from 0 to 100. A higher score means a better perceived health status.

share of voice (or share of noise)

The percentage of total promotional weight in a product category controlled by a particular company competing in that category. In practical terms in the pharmaceutical industry, share of voice might be defined by such criteria as number of details to target physicians compared with number of details by competitive sales forces.

side effects

Term for reactions to a drug other than the primary therapeutic one intended. Side effects may be negative, neutral, or positive. Some experts use side effects for relatively unimportant negative effects and adverse effects for more serious ones.

signs

Objective evidence of a disease or condition. Signs are disease manifestations that can be seen by the diagnostician and/or objectively measured. Symptoms, by contrast, are subjective manifestations that the diagnostician only learns of through patient self-report.

single-use devices (SUDs)

Medical devices that the manufacturer recommends be disposed of after just one use, such as syringes, surgical drills, and hemodialysis blood tubing. Increasingly, in an effort to control costs, purchasers such as hospitals have become interested in sterilization and reuse of such products (an activity known as reprocessing).

single-source products

Classification for drugs whose active ingredient is patent-protected. During that patent life, only one pharmaceutical company has a right to manufacture a product that contains that AI.

sizing

Determining the optimal number of sales representatives or account managers to support a brand or portfolio of brands.

skilled nursing care

Nursing services that can only be performed by or under the supervision of a registered nurse, such tube feeding and changing of sterile dressings. Any service that a layman could perform safely without RN supervision is not considered skilled care. Such services are available around the clock and are in accord with a physician's treatment orders. Some people need skilled care for a short time after an acute illness, while others require extended support. Skilled nursing is available in a variety of settings, including hospitals, SNFs, and even patient homes.

skilled nursing facility

See SNF.

SKU (stock-keeping unit)

A unique number assigned to a product for inventory and billing purposes. A single product usually has multiple SKUs assigned-each distinct color, size, flavor, or package requires a separate SKU to distinguish it.

site

In the pharmaceutical industry context, the place where subjects will see the investigator during a clinical trial. A single hospital, clinic, or other facility participating in a clinical trial.

site coordinator

A key member of the clinical team who works directly for the investigator at a particular site. Responsibilities usually include maintaining accurate patient documentation and dispensing medication. Sometimes referred to as the study coordinator or clinical research coordinator.

site initiation

A visit by a representative from the clinical trial sponsor (typically, the clinical research associate, also known as the monitor) to each site selected to participate in the upcoming trial. This meeting focuses on trial recruitment procedures and administrative preparations for the trial. The study protocol and the principal investigator's responsibilities under that protocol are also discussed.

small molecule

A term used to refer to drugs that are non-biologic (that is, chemical) in nature.

smart drugs

Drugs designed more precisely to minimize any impact other than the desired therapeutic one-which, therefore, have fewer side effects. Developing such drugs is one goal of biotechnology.

SMO (site management organization)

A company that specializes in the marketing and management of clinical development (clinical trials) services. Clinical trial sites (AMCs and IDNs) sometimes hire these vendors rather than building clinical development management and marketing capabilities in-house.

SNDA (Supplemental New Drug Application)

An application related to a drug for which the FDA has already approved the NDA, in which a request is made for approval of changes in packaging, labeling, dosages, ingredients, or indications.

SNF (skilled nursing facility)

Pronounced "sniff." An institution that provides specialized care (skilled nursing and/or relatively low-intensity rehabilitation) on an inpatient basis to people whose health status has stabilized. SNFs are an alternative to extended hospital stays or home care. Because patient acuity is relatively low, physician involvement in care is limited (e.g., to monthly visits).

SNP (single nucleotide polymorphism)

Pronounced "snip." A place in the genetic code at which significant variation in DNA sequence exists from person to person. These genetic differences are of interest because people with a specific variation may have a higher risk of a particular disease or be more responsive to a specific treatment.

source data

All information contained in original records such as patient charts, physician notes, and lab results. During clinical trials, such data are transferred to the case report form (CRF) for each trial subject.

source documents

Original records such as patient charts, physician notes, and lab results. During clinical trials, data from such records transferred to the case report form (CRF) for each trial subject.

sourcing

A function in pharmaceutical companies that controls decisions regarding whether it is appropriate to use outside vendors (including consultants) to perform a service or deliver a product–and, if so, on what terms contracting is permissible.

SPD (specialty pharmacy distributor)

A distributor whose products are limited to a relatively narrow category (e.g., biologic injectables, cancer drugs).

speaker programs

Conferences and meetings at which experts discuss topics of clinical or practical interest to pharmaceutical company customers. The pharmaceutical company may sponsor the conference or meeting as a promotional device to enhance relationships with the relevant customers (usually physicians and their office staff).

specialist

A physician with advanced training in a highly specific area of medicine, such as a cardiologist or oncologist. In some health plans, specialists cannot be seen without a referral from a gatekeeper physician, such as a general or family practitioner or internist.

specialty

The particular type of medical or surgical practice for which a physician is qualified.

specialty hospital

A hospital that concentrates on just one (typically complex) therapeutic area. The three primary categories are cardiac/heart hospitals, orthopedic hospitals, and spine hospitals.

specialty pharma

One (relatively narrow) definition: A company without an internal discovery engine that obtains all its products via in-licensing of drugs already on the market or in late-stage development. Typically, these products come from large pharmaceutical companies that do not want to invest their resources in marketing them (either due to limited sales potential or poor fit with current therapeutic focus).

The term is unfortunately used in a number of other, sometimes contradictory ways-to mean (a) emerging (early-stage) pharmaceutical companies; (b) generics, biotech, and drug delivery companies; (c) companies targeting niche markets; or (d) any entity that is neither a biotech nor Big Pharma.

specialty pharmacies

A niche pharmacy sector focused on people with chronic conditions, high drug costs, and complex care issues to be managed. Typical areas of specialization include cancer, hemophilia, HIV/AIDS, multiple sclerosis, infertility, rheumatoid arthritis, and biotech injectables.

Specialty pharmacies assume a more prominent role in care management than generalist pharmacies, helping payers to control costs for these expensive case types by encouraging patients understand and adhere to their prescribed therapy regimens.

specialty products

Diverse group of medications used in the management of uncommon illnesses that are typically prescribed by specialists rather than primary care physicians. Many specialty products are injectables.

specialty sales force

A sales force that promotes products that are used primarily by specialists.

specificity

The degree to which a drug produces acts in only one way on the body. Drugs with low specificity have many unintended effects. Selectivity refers to site of action; specificity concerns activity of the drug at a particular site.

In the realm of diagnostic testing, specificity means the ability to avoid "false positives"–identification of people without a disease as having the disease.

specification

For patents, the description of the invention for which a patent is being sought. This description is an essential part of the patent filing.

specifications

Criteria to which an intermediate or active pharmaceutical ingredient must conform to be considered acceptable for its intended use.

spend

Synonym for expenditure.

sponsor

The individual, company, or organization taking responsibility for initiation, management, and financing of a study. In the pharmaceutical context, the sponsor is often a pharmaceutical company, but it may be an individual, government agency, or academic or scientific institution.

SSRIs (selective serotonin reuptake inhibitors)

A category of drugs that are a prominent treatment for depression.

stability

A drug's resistance to change in physical and chemical properties (essential if it is to be stored for considerable periods of time before utilization).

staff-model HMO

The most restrictive type of HMO in terms of utilization controls, network size, and limits on use of outside providers. In this arrangement, most network physicians are salaried employees of the HMO; as a result of the employer-employee relationship, the HMO can rigorously managed physician utilization practices (diagnostic and therapeutic choices, including drug selection).

The HMO also owns most care settings in its networks, such as hospitals and physician office buildings. Patients must use, or bear heavy financial consequences for failing to use, "in network" physicians and institutions. Each practice site in a staff-model HMO typically includes a pharmacy, although the HMO may contract with community-based pharmacies as well to offer members greater convenience.

stage-gate process

A robust, well-defined process for analyzing opportunities. It includes decision points ("gates") at which standardized criteria are applied to make "go/no go" decisions. In the pharmaceutical context, a stage-gate process may be used to assess the potential of in-house compounds and outside products available for licensing.

standard drugs

A category used by FDA in defining priorities for NDA review. Standard drugs promise only modest (if any) improvement on drugs already on the market and/or do not treat a life-threatening disease; the FDA therefore accords their review lower priority and sets a 10-month NDA review turnaround goal. By contrast, see priority drugs, which the FDA tries to review within just 6 months.

standard operating procedure (SOP)

Official, detailed, written instructions for the management of clinical trials or the manufacturing of a drug formulation.

Stark I and II

Federal laws whose combined effect is to prohibit any physician from referring Medicare or Medicaid patients to entities in which the physician or an immediate family member of the physician has an ownership interest or with which the physician or family member has some type of compensation arrangement.

Although Stark is referred to as a law against self-referral (that is, referral to an entity in which one has a financial stake), it applies more broadly to other arrangements in which a physician is financially rewarded for generating service or product sales. Stark I limited the prohibition to clinical laboratories. Stark II extended the prohibition to other "designated health services," including outpatient prescription drugs.

The Stark law has a number of safe harbor exceptions, which include:
- Receipt by a physician of items of negligible value
- Fair market value compensation for services actually rendered by the physician
- Discounts on drug prices, so long as:
  - The same discount is offered to other similarly situated physicians
  - The same discount is offered to other similarly situated physicians
  - The discount is not tied to volume of the drug ordered
  - The full benefit of the discount is passed on to the insurer

See Anti-kickback.

statistically powered

Involving a sample sufficiently large to reveal statistically significant differences.

stem cell

An undifferentiated cell with the potential to become any type of special-ized cell. Most embryo cells are stem cells. They might provide an unlimited source of healthy adult cells, such as bone, muscle, liver, or blood, to treat people with various diseases. Stem cells are already used as therapies for blood disorders and some forms of cancer.

step therapy

The practice of beginning treatment with most cost-effective drug therapy and progressing to more expensive and/or risky therapy only if the initial treatment is unsuccessful.

steroid

Member of a large family of structurally similar lipid substances, but differ-ent classes of steroids have different functions. For instance, all the natural sex hormones are steroids. Anabolic steroids increase muscle mass, while anti-inflammatory steroids (also known as corticosteroids) can reduce swelling, pain, and other manifestations of inflammation.

structural genomics

The use of 3-D models of genomes known or suspected to play a role in a particular disease/condition. Based on the model, researchers try to identify compounds that will interact the protein target to produce a health benefit.

structure-activity relationship (SAR)

The effect of a drug's chemical makeup on its pharmacological behavior (activity). Molecular structure and activity are correlated by modifying the structure and observing the impact on defined endpoints.

structure-guided drug discovery

Use of proprietary technologies for quickly identifying the structure of target genes or proteins, which expedites the creation of chemicals (drugs) to address maladies associated with those target structures.

study coordinator

A person (often a nurse) responsible for many aspects of study administration at a particular site, including completion of case report forms. Study coordinators often serve as liaisons between the study sponsor and the site. Also known as a clinical research coordinator or study nurse.

study monitors

Sponsor personnel who visit trial sites regularly to ensure protocol adherence and check the reliability and completeness of data collected.

subacute care

Short-term care provided by many long-term care facilities and hospitals for patients who no longer need acute care services but are not yet ready for discharge to their homes.

subject

A participant in a clinical trial.

supplements

Defined in the Dietary Supplement Health and Education Act (DSHEA) of 1994 as a product taken by mouth that contains a "dietary ingredient" intended to provide nutritional value. The "dietary ingredients" in these products may include vitamins, minerals, herbs or other botanicals, amino acids, and substances such as enzymes and metabolites. They are available as everything from pills and powders to nutrition bars.

DSHEA made dietary supplements a subcategory of foods, not drugs. As a result, supplements are now subject to far less rigorous regulation than pharmaceuticals or even foods. The FDA has not defined manufacturing standards for supplements as yet; supplements do not need prior approval from the FDA to be marketed in the US; and unless the supplement contains a new dietary ingredient, the seller does not need to provide evidence of safety or efficacy to the FDA either before or after it begins marketing the product. The manufacturers and distributors are not even required to report adverse events to the FDA. Once a supplement is on the market, the FDA can only intervene to restrict its use after showing that the drug is actually unsafe.

supply chain

The series of activities involved in drug manufacture and sale, from resource and facilities procurement through distribution.

suppression

Elimination or prevention of manifestations (signs or symptoms) of a disease. Suppression treatment may be necessary over the entire lifetime of a person with a chronic disease.

In the context of organ transplants, suppression involves the use of drugs to avert an immune response by the body to the foreign tissue.

surrogate endpoint (or surrogate marker)

A laboratory finding or physical sign that does not directly signal an improvement in (or stabilization of) a patient's mental or physical health, functioning, or survival rate, but is considered a likely indicator of such improvement. For instance, in patients with a history of heart disease, a reduction in a risk factor such as "bad" cholesterol levels would be considered a surrogate endpoint. Tumor regression is a surrogate endpoint in cancer trials.

Surrogate markers are often used when the length of time required to assess such direct indicators of efficacy as survival rates is prohibitively long.

When the FDA approves a drug based on surrogate markers alone, it then requires a post-marketing clinical trial to confirm actual clinical benefit.

surveillance studies

See post-market surveillance.

suspension

Drug packaged form where the active ingredient is mixed with a liquid, usually water, in which it cannot dissolve. As a result, the active ingredient remains intact in the form of tiny particles.

sustained release

A delivery mechanism that dispenses a drug in the body gradually, ensuring a steady level in the blood and relatively long-term effect. Sustained-release products can be administered less frequently than those that are metabolized more quickly. Sometimes referred to as extended release.

switching

Changing over from a previously utilized drug to a new one for the same condition, risk factor (e.g., high cholesterol), or disease.

symptoms

Subjective sensations related to a disease or condition. Symptoms are indicators that the diagnostician learns about only through patient self-report. By contrast, signs are manifestations that can be seen by the diagnostician and/or objectively measured.

synergism

The combined action of two or more chemicals (or drugs), which results in an effect that is greater than the sum of their effects taken independently.

synthesis

The production of a substance (e.g., as in protein synthesis) through the combination of chemical elements, groups, or simpler compounds, or by the breaking down of a complex compound.

synthetic drugs

Drugs that are created in laboratories, as opposed to drugs that are endogenous (originating or produced within an organism, tissue, or cell). Many antibiotics, such as amoxicillin and ampicillin, are considered semi-synthetic drugs, as they are a form of pencillin, which itself is not synthetic. Amphetamine, on the other hand, is a wholly synthetic drug.

systems biology

The study of interactions among various elements of biological systems (including, but not limited to, genes and proteins). One practical use is identifying targets for new drug development.

systolic pressure

The higher of the two readings obtained when blood pressure is measured. The systole is the period when the chambers of the heart contract, and blood is pumped into the arteries.

T

target

Compounds in the body, usually proteins, whose action or inaction is related to a disease or condition. Once a target associated with a disease is identified, a company can attempt to develop drugs that affect its operation. Receptors and enzymes are two very common types of target.

target profile

A set of ideal characteristics for a product in development, based on the characteristics that would enhance its performance and marketability.

target validation

The process of proving that a drug/compound interacting with a specific target associated with a disease produces a health benefit. In a sense, the more appropriate term might be drug validation.

target universe

In the pharmaceutical context, the group of physicians or specialties (e.g., GPs and internists) identified as likely prescribers of drugs for a specific indication. Within that target universe, pharmaceutical company sales forces may concentrate solely on physicians likely to be high prescribers.

teaching hospital

A hospital with an accredited medical residency training program. Such hospitals are typically affiliated with a medical school.

teratogenic

Causing abnormal fetal development.

tertiary care

Highly specialized medical and surgical care for unusual or complex medical problems provided by a large medical center, usually serving a region or state and having highly sophisticated technological and support facilities.

test group

The group in a controlled clinical trial receiving the investigational drug or treatment that the study is designed to evaluate.

therapeutic (or therapy) area

A clinical discipline. Therapeutic areas include the basic internal medicine specialties (cardiology, gastroenterology, rheumatology, and nephrology, for example), as well as such other disciplines as psychiatry, neurology, oncology, infectious disease, and anesthesiology. Many pharmaceutical companies organize functions within R&D by therapeutic area. Sales figures for pharmaceutical products by therapy area provide pharmaceutical marketers with a useful index of the commercial market.

therapeutic category

A system of grouping drugs by common therapeutic indication. Generally speaking, a less-broad grouping than therapeutic area. Hundreds of different categorization systems exist.

One example, the American Hospital Formulary System, assigns a 6-digit classification code that combines category, class, and subclass. For instance, in the classification 08:12.04, the "08" stands for the category, anti-infective agents; the "12" for the class, antibiotics; and the "04" for the subclass, antifungal agents.

therapeutic class

Drugs that share both an indication and a method of operation. For instance, ACE (angiotensin-converting enzyme) inhibitors are a class of drugs that treat high blood pressure by inhibiting a particular enzyme.

A narrower grouping than therapeutic category. Therapeutic class and drug class are synonyms.

When a new class of drug emerges to treat a disease, the challenge for pharmaceutical companies begins not at the brand level but at the therapeutic-class level-convincing potential prescribers that this new approach will be effective.

therapeutic equivalents

Two drugs that are roughly interchangeable in safety and efficacy when used at roughly the same dose to treat the same health problem.

In compiling the Orange Book, the FDA uses the term solely for drugs with the same active ingredient(s), not for drugs with different active ingredients that are used to treat the same condition.

therapeutics

Drugs used to treat one or more diseases or conditions.

therapeutic index

A measure of drug safety; a drug with a high index is considered safer than one with a low index.

therapeutic substitution

The replacement of the drug prescribed by a physician with another prescription brand (rather than a generic) that is believed to produce an equally good health result. The drug substituted is usually, but not always, in the same drug class as the one originally prescribed. Therapeutic substitution is most common in hospitals, where the P&T Committee may make a "blanket ruling" to change all physician prescriptions for one brand to another brand that is considered equivalent (and often less expensive).

therapeutic window

The dosage range at which a drug is both safe and efficacious.

Alternatively, the time period during which a drug or other treatment can be expected to have a beneficial effect if administered. A narrow therapeutic window means that the drug must be administered relatively soon after the onset of symptoms to be effective.

third-party administrator (TPA)

A services provider or insurance company that processes claims on behalf of a self-insured organization. The administrator is considered a third party because it is neither the self-insurer (often an employer) nor an insured recipient of health services (often an employee).

third-party payer (TPP)

A public or private organization that pays or insures health or medical expenses on behalf of beneficiaries or recipients. For example, the federal government is a third-party payer under Medicare.

thought leaders

See key opinion leaders (KOLs).

TIA (transient ischemic attack)

A minor stroke with symptoms such as temporary loss of speech or paralysis of an arm or leg. These symptoms abate within 24 hours.

tiered formularies

System employed by many MCOs to encourage use of preferred rather than non-preferred drugs. Formularies typically have three "grades," from most favored (Tier I) to least favored (Tier III). The most-favored drugs are usually inexpensive generics, which carry the lowest co-payments as an incentive for members to choose them. Favored brands are typically assigned to Tier II. Differences in co-payments based on tier vary from modest to quite substantial.

tissue

Section of an organ that consists of a largely homogenous population of cell types.

titration

Gradual increases/decreases in drug dose until a desired clinical effect is achieved.

tolerability

The ability of a patient to remain on therapy despite any adverse or side effects associated with it. Drugs that patients rarely stop taking due to such effects are considered well tolerated.

tolerance

Increase in body's resistance to the effects of a drug, leading to the need for higher doses to produce the same benefits.

topical product

A medication applied to body surfaces such as the skin or mucous membranes (e.g., vagina, nasopharynx, eye). Examples include ointments, creams, gels, and lotions. Topical medications should not be confused with transdermal medications, which achieve their effect by being absorbed through the skin.

toxic effects

Extremely serious adverse effects.

toxicity

The degree to which a drug or other substance is poisonous to an animal or person.

Also, the actual occurrence of adverse events in people taking the drug. The level of acceptable toxicity will vary depending on the condition a drug is used to treat.

toxicology

Division of medical and biological science concerned with the study of the harmful effects of various substances, including drugs.

TPA

See third-party administrator.

In the context of cardiovascular health, TPA (or tPA) means tissue plasminogen activator-a drug used to break up the blood clots that are the leading cause of both strokes and heart attacks. It is often used to prevent recurrence in people who have already suffered either a heart attack or stroke.

trade

Pharmaceutical company customer segment that includes wholesalers and retail pharmacies.

trade name

The name that a pharmaceutical company gives a product for promotional purposes, in order to differentiate it from others in the marketplace. Patented drugs are usually sold under a trade name. Generic versions manufactured after expiration of a patent may be sold under either the generic name (for example, ibuprofen) or a trade name (for example, Motrin). A trade name is also referred to as a brand name.

trauma center

An emergency room that is equipped and staffed to care for serious traumatic injuries.

treatment

Alleviation of symptoms of chronic diseases and (sometimes) reduction in the risk of disease progression.

treatment arm or treatment group

In a clinical trial, a group of participants who all receive the same treatment (i.e., investigational drug, comparator drug, or placebo).

treatment protocol

Step-by-step guidelines specifying the optimal therapy regimen for a specific disease or condition. Also referred to as a treatment algorithm.

Treatment IND (TIND)

A means used by the FDA to make promising new drugs available as early in the development process as possible to desperately or seriously ill patients who have no treatment alternative. The FDA grants TIND status based on preliminary evidence of effectiveness. Drugs given TIND approval are utilized primarily for actual treatment, rather than to test a drug's safety and efficacy in clinical trials.

Treatment INDs, along with Emergency INDs, are known as Compassionate INDs (although the term "Compassionate" is not specified in the IND regulations).

triple option plan

A combined health plan that offers enrollees the choice of an HMO, PPO, or indemnity insurance. In contrast to POS arrangements, enrollees must choose among those options at the point of enrollment rather than ad hoc for each episode of care.

tumor specificity

The extent to which a chemotherapy agent can attack cancer cells without damaging non-malignant cells, such as those in the gastrointestinal tract and bone marrow. It is very important to develop new chemotherapeutic agents with improved tumor specificity.

Tx

Shorthand for treatment.

U

UCR (usual, customary, and reasonable)

The standard employed by insurers to define how much they will pay a provider for a given service under a fee-for-service system. If the provider charges a higher fee for that service, it will either go unpaid (because the contract between provider and plan states that the consumer will not have to pay any differential) or the patient will be responsible for making up the difference.

unbranded Web site

A Web site built by a pharmaceutical company prior to the launch of a new brand. An unbranded Web site serves two purposes:

- Informing consumers (and physicians) about the disease state (thus raising disease awareness and encouraging diagnosis of affected consumers)
- Establishing the pharmaceutical company as the trusted information resource for the disease or condition the drug will treat

United States Pharmacopeial Convention

A nonprofit, nongovernmental standards-setting organization that advances public health by ensuring the quality and consistency of medicines, promoting the safe and proper use of medications, and verifying ingredients in dietary supplements. Its publications are described under USP.

upcoding

Assigning a care episode a billing code that carries higher reimbursement than the appropriate one for the treatment provided. Deliberate upcoding is considered fraud.

uptake

In clinical terms, the absorption and incorporation of a substance by living tissue-in the pharmaceutical context, a drug by the human body. Many drugs have relatively rapid uptake into the bloodstream, but must be administered repeatedly to continue providing health benefits.

In commercial terms, the rate at which a product is adopted by prescribers, payers, and the relevant patient population. Pharmaceutical companies need to anticipate how quickly use will increase following a product's introduction in order to project market potential. That is, a product that will reach its peak sales target in six months will be more profitable than one that will take two years to reach peak sales, even if the peak number is the same for both products.

USAN (US Adopted Name)

The nonproprietary (generic) name assigned to a new chemical entity by the US Adopted Names Council, a private organization sponsored by the American Medical Association, the United States Pharmacopeia, and the American Pharmaceutical Association.

USP (United States Pharmacopeia)

A variety of publications from the United States Pharmacopeial Convention that explain the uses and purity standards for drugs.

A three-volume reference work covering both generic and ethical drug products, United States Pharmacopoeia-DI, explains their appropriate uses.

The United States Pharmacopeia and National Formulary (USP-NF) provides standards of identity, strength, quality, and purity for prescription and non-prescription drug ingredients and dosage forms, dietary supplements, medical devices, and other healthcare products. It includes tests, analytical procedures, and acceptance criteria.

USPTO

The regulatory agency that grants US patents for concepts that are both unique and useful. Among other things, the PTO grants US patents to pharmaceutical companies for drugs, other "manufactures," and key processes.

utilization review (UR)

Evaluation by a health plan or healthcare institution of the cost-efficacy of care decisions made by a group of physicians. DUR, or drug utilization review, is a subcategory of evaluations of resource use.

Utilization review may be either retrospective (after the resources have been used) or prospective (for instance, pre-authorization requirements).

V

VA

Department of Veterans Affairs, the federal agency that provides eligible US veterans with medical care and operates a network of VA hospitals. Part of the Federal Markets customer segment. See VHA.

vaccine

A biologic that the immune system recognizes as a disease-causing agent. The antibodies produced by the body as a result protect the body against a more serious attack by the same antigen. Some vaccines, such as for smallpox and polio, have essentially eliminated these diseases from the US and many parts of the world

validated facilities

FDA-approved drug manufacturing sites.

validated target

A drug target (typically a protein) that has been proven to have an effect on human health. Therefore, interventions affecting that target have therapeutic potential.

validation

Documentary proof offered by a drug manufacturer to the FDA that its manu-facturing processes will produce the same drug product batch to batch and year to year.

value proposition

A compelling definition, for marketing purposes, of the advantages of using a certain drug-in terms of clinical efficacy, safety, convenience, and/or health-care-related cost savings for payers and patients.

variable co-pays

Differences in out-of-pocket costs for patients/consumers, employed by MCOs to discourage use of costly or disfavored pharmaceuticals. Variable co-payments are part of tiered formulary arrangements. Typically, the co-pay is higher if the drug is a brand with a lower-cost generic equivalent, is not a preferred one on the formulary, or is not on the formulary at all.

ventilator

A breathing machine. Also called a respirator.

vertical integration

Consolidation or merger of organizations that provide a continuum of related services. In the healthcare context, that might mean a health system acquiring physician practices and a nursing home.

VHA (Veterans Health Administration)

The division within the Department of Veterans Affairs charged with providing medical care to eligible US veterans. A target customer for the pharmaceutical company Managed Markets function. Part of Federal Markets.

virus

Minute infectious agents (much smaller than bacteria). Viruses, which can replicate only within living host cells, cause many types of illness.

W-Z

warning letter

The most serious form of citation letter from the FDA to a pharmaceutical company regarding regulatory problems such as misleading promotional communications or inadequate manufacturing controls.

WBC (white blood cell)

A type of blood cell that helps the body fight infection and disease. These cells originate in the bone marrow and then travel to other parts of the body. Also known as a leukocyte.

wellness

Programs aimed at promoting healthier lifestyles and identifying people at risk for certain diseases, in order to reduce healthcare costs via early behavioral change and treatment intervention.

WHO (World Health Organization)

The United Nations health agency, founded to enhance the health of people around the world. It makes recommendations regarding practices countries should adopt to control diseases. WHO coordinates responses to major epidemics, particularly in developing countries.

wholesale acquisition cost (WAC)

The price a wholesaler pays when purchasing drugs from a manufacturer, not taking into account any discounts.

wholesalers

Entities that purchase drugs from pharmaceutical companies and then resell and deliver them to pharmacies. Pharmaceutical companies often collaborate with wholesalers to monitor demand and ensure product availability in the marketplace.

withdrawal

FDA rescission of approval for marketing a drug or other product in the US. Once the FDA has approved a product, it can only be withdrawn based on a finding that it is no longer safe or effective.

When safety or effectiveness issues arise, pharmaceutical companies often work cooperatively with the FDA to make labeling changes or, if necessary, execute a voluntary withdrawal of the product from the market. The arthritis and acute pain medication Vioxx was voluntarily withdrawn from the market by Merck & Co. when results of a clinical trial revealed significant safety issues with the drug. The FDA may also request that a company "voluntarily" withdraw its product from the market, as it did with Pfizer's NSAID Bextra.

World Trade Organization (WTO)

The international organization dealing with global commerce, which address-es trade-related aspects of intellectual property rights to drugs. In its role as an advocate for poorer nations, it has negotiated with pharmaceutical companies to obtain free or discounted drugs and permission for those countries to use generic versions of still-patented drugs.

21 CFR Part 11

Known as the Electronic Record Rule. FDA standards set forth in the Code of Federal Regulations concerning use of electronic (rather than paper-based) records and signatures.

Abbeviations and Acronyms

AAC
Actual acquisition cost

AACP
American Association of Colleges of Pharmacy

AAHP
American Association of Health Plans

AAPS
American Association of Pharmaceutical Scientists

Ab
Antibody

ABX
Antibiotics

ACCP
American College of Clinical Pharmacy

ACE
Adverse clinical event or angiotensin–converting enzyme (inhibitor)

ADDAT
Average daily dose after titration

ADE
Adverse drug event

ADHD
Attention deficit/hyperactivity disorder

ADI
Acceptable daily intake

ADL
Activities of daily living

ADME
Absorption, distribution, metabolism, and excretion

ADR
Adverse drug reaction

AE
Adverse event

AERS
Adverse event reporting system

AHA
American Hospital Association

AHCPR
Agency for Health Care Policy and Research

AHRQ
Agency for Healthcare Research and Quality

AK
Actinic keratosis

AIDS
Acquired immunodeficiency syndrome

AIM
Active ingredient manufacturer

ALF
Assisted living facility

ALOS
Average length of stay

ALS
Amyotrophic lateral sclerosis (Lou Gehrig's disease)

AM
Account manager

AMA
American Medical Association OR American Marketing Association

AMC
Academic medical center

AML
Acute myeloid leukemia

AMP
Average manufacturer's price

ANA
American Nurses Association

ANDA
Abbreviated New Drug Application

APCs
Ambulatory Payment Classifications

APhA
American Pharmaceutical Association

API
Active pharmaceutical ingredient

APLB
Advertising and Promotional Labeling Branch

ARB
Angiotensin-receptor blocker

ASC
Ambulatory surgery center

ASCPT
American Society for Clinical Pharmacy and Therapeutics

ASHP
American Society of Health-System Pharmacists

ASO
Administrative services only

AWP
Average wholesale price

BCBS
Blue Cross Blue Shield

BD
Business Development or twice daily

BID or bid
Twice daily (on prescriptions)

BIND
Biologic investigational new drug

BIO
Biotechnology Industry Organization

BLA
Biologic license application

BMI
Body mass index

BMJ
British Medical Journal

BMT
Bone marrow transplant

BP
Blood pressure

CABG
Coronary artery bypass graft

CAC
Carrier advisory committee

CAD
Coronary artery disease

CADD
Computer-assisted drug design

CAMP
Consortium for the Advancement of Manufacturing for Pharmaceuticals

CAT
Computerized axial tomography (scan)

CBC
Complete blood count

CBER
Center for Biologics Evaluation and Research (within FDA)

CCRC
Certified clinical research coordinator

CCU
Coronary care unit

CDC
Centers for Disease Control and Prevention

CDER
Center for Drug Evaluation and Research (within FDA)

CF
Cystic fibrosis

CFR
Code of Federal Regulations

cGMP
Current good manufacturing practices

CHD
Coronary or congenital heart disease

CHF
Congestive heart failure

CKD
Chronic kidney disease

CMC
Chemistry, manufacturing, and controls

CME
Continuing medical education

CMO
Contract manufacturing organization

CMS
Centers for Medicare and Medicaid Services (formerly HCFA)

CNM
Certified nurse midwife

CNP
Certified nurse practitioner

CNS
Central nervous system or clinical nurse specialist

COGS
Cost of goods sold

COPD
Chronic obstructive pulmonary disease

CPG
Clinical Program Guidance

CPMP
(European) Committee for Proprietary Medical Products

CPO
Contract pharmaceutical organization

CRA
Clinical research associate

CRC
Clinical research coordinator

CRF
Case report form

CRI
Chronic renal insufficiency

CRNA
Certified registered nurse anesthetist

CRO
Contract research organization

CRM
Customer relationship management

CSO
Contract sales organization

CT
Computerized tomography

CVA
Cerebrovascular incident (a stroke)

DALY
Disability adjusted life year

DAW
Dispense as written

DBP
Diastolic blood pressure

DDMAC
Division of Drug Marketing, Advertising and Communications (within the FDA)

DEA
Drug Enforcement Administration

DHHS
Department of Health and Human Services

DIA
Drug Information Association

DM
District manager (Sales) or diabetes mellitus

DMARD
Disease-modifying antirheumatic drug

DME
Durable medical equipment

DMR
Direct member reimbursement

DNA
Deoxyribonucleic acid

DO
Doctor of osteopathy

Department of Defense
Department of Defense

DoJ
Department of Justice

DRG
Diagnosis-related group

DS
Down syndrome

DSHEA
Dietary Supplement Health and Education Act

DSM
District Sales Manager

DTC
Direct to consumer (advertising)

DTP
Direct to physician (advertising)

DPR
Drug price review

DUR
Drug utilization review

Dx
Diagnosis

ECHO
Economic, clinical, and humanistic outcomes

ED
Emergency department or erectile dysfunction

EFPIA
European Federation of Pharmaceutical Industries and Associations

EMEA
European Medicines Evaluation Agency

ENT
Ear, nose, and throat

EMR
Electronic medical record

EOP
End of phase

EPL
Effective patent life

EPO
Exclusive provider organization or erythropoietin

ERISA
Employee Retirement Income Security Act of 1974

ESRD
End-stage renal disease

FCP
Federal ceiling price

FDA
Food and Drug Administration

FDAMA
FDA Modernization Act of 1997

FDCA
Federal Food, Drug, and Cosmetic Act of 1938

FEBHP
Federal Employees Health Benefits Program

FFS
Fee for service

FP
Family practitioner

FSA
Flexible spending account

FSS
Federal Supply Schedule

FTC
Federal Trade Commission

FTIM
First time in man

GCP
Good clinical practice

GFR
Glomular filtration rate

GI
Gastrointestinal

GLP
Good laboratory practice

GMP
Good manufacturing practice

GP
General practitioner

GPhA or GPIA
Generic Pharmaceutical Association or Generic Pharmaceutical Industry Association

GPO
Group purchasing organization

Hb
Hemoglobin

HBV
Hepatitis B virus

HCFA
Health Care Financing Administration (now known as CMS)

HCT
Hematocrit

HCV
Hepatitis C virus

HD
Hemodialysis or Hodgkin's disease (lymphoma)

HDL
High-density lipoprotein

HDMA
Health Distribution Management Association

HEDIS
Health Employer Data and Information Set

Hgb
Hemoglobin

HHC
Home healthcare

HHS
Health and Human Services

HIPAA
Health Insurance Portability and Accountability Act of 1996

HIV
Human immunodeficiency virus

HL-7
Health Level Seven

HMO
Health maintenance organization

HPLC
High-performance liquid chromatography

HRA
Health reimbursement account

HRT
Hormone replacement therapy

HSA
Health savings account

Hx
History

IBS
Irritable bowel syndrome

ICD-9
International Classification of Diseases, Ninth Revision

ICH
International Council on Harmonization

ICU
Intensive care unit

IDN
Integrated delivery network

IND
Investigational new drug or investigational new drug application

INDA
Investigational new drug application

IP
Intellectual property

IPA
Independent practice association

IRB
Institutional review board

JAMA
Journal of the American Medical Association

KOL
Key opinion leader

LCA
Least costly alternative

LDL
Low-density lipoprotein

LESI
Licensing Executives Society International

LMRP
Local medical review policy

LOS
Length of stay

LPN
Licensed practical nurse

LTC
Long-term care

MA
Medical Affairs

MAbs
Monoclonal antibodies

MAC
Maximum allowable cost

MBHO
Managed behavioral health organization

MCO
Managed care organization

MDC
Major Diagnostic Category

Mg/dL
Milligrams per deciliter

MI
Myocardial infarction

ml
Milliliter

MLHW
Ministry of Health, Labor, and Welfare

MMA
Medical Marketing Association

MMO
Managed markets organization

MMR
Measles, mumps, and rubella

MOA
Mechanism of action

MOAbs
Monoclonal antibodies

MPPPA
Medicaid Prudent Pharmaceutical Purchasing Act of 1990

MRI
Magnetic resonance imaging

mRNA
Messenger RNA

MS
Multiple sclerosis

MSL
Medical science liaison

MTD
Maximum tolerated dose

M+C

Medicare Plus Choice

M&M

Morbidity and mortality

NABP

National Association of Boards of Pharmacy

NACDS

National Association of Chain Drug Stores

NAM

National account manager

NCD

National coverage determination

NCE

New chemical entity

NCPA

National Community Pharmacists Association

NCPDP

National Council for Prescription Drug Programs

NCQA

National Committee for Quality Assurance

NCS

National Cancer Society

NDA
New drug application

NDC
National Drug Code

NEJM
New England Journal of Medicine

NF
National formulary

NHL
Non-Hodgkin's lymphoma

NIA
National Institute on Aging

NICU
Neonatal intensive care unit

NIH
National Institutes of Health

NIMH
National Institute of Mental Health

NINDS
National Institute of Neurological Disorders and Stroke

NOC
Notice of compliance

NOV
Notice of violation

NP
Nurse practitioner

NME
New molecular entity

NPO
Nil per os (nothing by mouth)

NSAID
Non-steroidal anti-inflammatory drug

NTI
Narrow therapeutic index or nonthyroidal illness

NWDA
National Wholesale Druggists Association

OA
Osteoarthritis

OCD
Obsessive-compulsive disorder

OIG
Office of Inspector General

OPPS
Outpatient Prospective Payment System

OTC
Over the counter

PA
Physician assistant

PAR
Post-approval research

PAT
Process Analytical Technologies

PBM
Pharmacy benefit manager

PCP
Primary care physician or practitioner

PCR
Polymerase chain reaction

PD
Peritoneal dialysis or pharmacodynamics or Parkinson's disease

PDA
Personal digital assistant

PDL
Preferred drug list

PDMA
Prescription Drug Marketing Act of 1987

PDR
Physicians' Desk Reference

PDUFA
Prescription Drug User Fee Act of 1992

PET
Positron emission tomography (scan)

PGx
Pharmacogenomics

pH
Hydrogen ion concentration (acid-base scale)

PHO
Physician-hospital organization

PhRMA
Pharmaceutical Research and Manufacturers of America

PHS
Public Health Service

PI
Package insert or principal investigator

PK
Pharmacokinetics

PMA
Pre-market approval

PMPM
Per member per month

PMPY
Per member per year

PO
Per os (by mouth)

POA
Plan of action

POC
Proof of concept

POS
Point-of-service (plan)

PPM or PPMC
Physician practice management corporation

PPO
Preferred provider organization

PPS
Prospective payment service or plasma protein solution

PRN
Pro re nata (as needed)

PT
Physical therapy

Pt

Patient

PTCA

Percutaneous transvenous coronary angioplasty

PTO

US Patent and Trade Office

P&T

Pharmacy and Therapeutics (committee)

Px

Physical examination

P1

First product to be promoted (in a sales detail)

P2

Second product to be promoted (in a sales detail)

P3

Third product to be promoted (in a sales detail)

Q

Every (e.g., Q6h = every 6 hours)

QA

Quality assurance

QC

Quality control

Qd
Daily

Qh
Every hour

QID or qid
Four times a day

QOD
Every other day

QoL
Quality of life

QW
Every week

RA
Rheumatoid arthritis or Regulatory Affairs

RAM
Regional account manager (Managed Markets)

RBC
Red blood cell

RCT
Randomized clinical trial

rDNA
Recombinant DNA

RLD
Reference listed drug

RN
Registered nurse

RNA
Ribonucleic acid

RSD
Regional sales director

RT
Respiratory therapy or radiation therapy

RTI
Respiratory tract infection

RUG
Resource Utilization Group

Rx
Prescription

SAE
Serious adverse event

SAR
Structure-activity relationship

SARS
Severe acute respiratory syndrome

SC
Subcutaneous or study coordinator or site coordinator or sickle cell

SFA
Sales force automation

SFI
Sales force intelligence

SF-36
Short Form 36

SICU
Surgical intensive care unit

SIDS
Sudden infant death syndrome

SKU
Stock-keeping unit

SMO
Site management organization

SNDA
Supplemental New Drug Application

SNF
Skilled nursing facility

SNP
Single nucleotide polymorphism

SOP
Standard operating procedure

SPD
Specialty pharmacy distributor

SSRI
Selective serotonin reuptake inhibitor

STD
Sexually transmitted disease

SUD
Single-use device

Sx
Symptoms

THR
Total hip replacement

TIA
Transient ischemic attack

TDD
Total daily dose

TID or tid
Three times a day

TIND
Treatment investigational new drug

TNF
Tumor necrosis factor

TPA
Third-party administrator or tissue plasminogen activator

TPP
Third-party payer

TRx
Total prescriptions

TSH
Thyroid stimulating hormone

Tx
Treatment

UR
Utilization review

URTI
Upper respiratory tract infection

USAN
United States Adopted Name

USP
United States Pharmacopeia

USP-NF
United States Pharmacopeia-National Formulary

USPTO
US Patent and Trademark Office

UTI
Urinary tract infection

VA
Veterans Administration (Department of Veterans Affairs)

VF
Ventricular failure or ventricular fibrillation

VHA
Veterans Health Administration

WAC
Wholesale acquisition cost

WBC
White blood cell

WHO
World Health Organization

WTO
World Trade Organization